Alzheimer's Wife

A Caregiver's Journey From Endurance to Resilience

B. Jensen

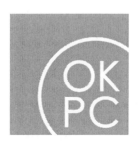

Published by:

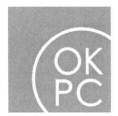

www.OKanaganPublishingCo.ca

Okanagan Publishing Co is an imprint of
Okanagan Publishing Inc
1024 Lone Pine Court
Kelowna, BC V1P 1M7
www.okanaganpublishinghouse.ca

Printed in the United States of America

1st Edition, March 2022

10   9   8   7   6   5   4   3   2   1

ISBN: 978-1-990389-07-8

"For in and out, above, about, below,

'Tis nothing but a Magic Shadow-show,

Play'd in a Box whose Candle is the Sun,

Round which we Phantom Figures come and go"

- Rubaiyat of Omar Khayyam, XLVI

CONTENTS

PART TWO: RESILIENCE

A Spider Metaphor

Many times, it seems that I am just aimlessly typing words. As soon as I recall something, I am stirred to write about it but the theme, scenes, characters, point of view and all the other things one needs to write well arrange themselves randomly as they please. Often there is little sense to what my mind conjures up. Yet, sometimes I succeed in reviving moments of joy and sorrow in reasonable paragraphs.

Recently a fascinating television documentary told of the life of spiders. I have admired their artistic and symmetrical webs; particularly when they are displayed against a green background, covered with dew and radiant with sunbeams caught in the moist strings. When a bird, a falling leaf or storm partially destroy the web, the awesome design and beauty disappear strand by strand. The spider rushes out and with innate skill repairs the damage. In quick time the splendor of his web reappears.

Somehow, I can look at the last eight years of my life as an *Alzheimer's Wife* in this way. I do not like the years of watching my husband's mind and body slowly, ever so slowly, disintegrating. In his case repairs cannot be made, but some strands of his life remain.

The glimmer of a smile in his eyes reminds me of the many hours I have gazed into their deep blue. I had been enchanted as they eagerly reached into my heart and passion. His laughter and touch had caught me yearning for more. Now his bright smiling eyes are almost closed and have lost their gleam. Now we only hold hands. These hands, that were once skilled, gentle and warm, are now gnarled, wrinkled and cold as I hold them in my warm ones. He was six feet tall. I always looked up at him with my five foot three inches. I had to stand on tiptoes to kiss him. Now I lean over him as he sits bent in his wheelchair or rests listlessly in his bed. I kiss him on his bald head which once was covered with rich, dark, wavy hair. His infectious grin is now only a feeble smile. His body that loved to move to music and all the rhythms of life is now unwilling to move without a lot of help.

In nature the spider does its work, always repairing his torn home. My husband and I had also created an intricate web. A web of marriage and family. Then in 2009, a strange spider appeared in our lives. A spider called Alzheimer's. He does not repair. That spider slowly, very slowly for the last twelve years, has been destroying the intricate web we had woven for over fifty years. Still, I keep thinking of how amazingly beautiful this web once was. Only tiny, shiny shreds remain and as I look at my husband today, they remind me of what once was. I try to shy away from the fact that they too will disappear, as the man, whom I have always loved, fades away. All I can do now is hope that my Darling will one day soon rest in peace.

PART ONE:

ENDURANCE

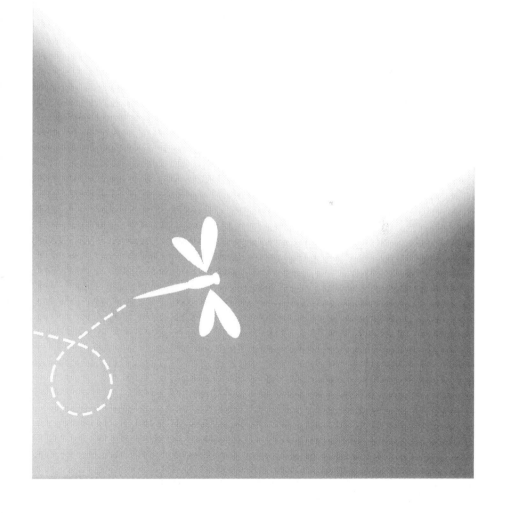

Chapter 1:

Long, Long Ago

I sit, many a morning, in my favourite chair on my balcony with that first cup of coffee of the day and let my mind wander.

These wanderings help me stay positive. Some memories are more than half a century old but remind me of better times, before sad events unfolded. When Alzheimer's entered our lives and immense challenges had to be met, I had to restructure my life completely.

This morning a fresh breeze is in the air, gentle but invigorating. My mind goes back to one special day during our honeymoon, sixty-one years ago in the springtime, when the day was also invigorating.

Kaj and I had visited a lush park outside of Copenhagen. Here, too, a fresh breeze wafted through the woods. The path curved around shrubs, flowerbeds, green meadows, and magnificent statues of important people of history. All of a sudden, Kaj grabbed my hand.

"Quick, come along." He laughed. "Let's see what is over there behind the trees."

We dashed off the path into the woods and breathlessly stopped. I had no idea where we were or why we had stopped here. Then, suddenly, my handsome new husband held me in his arms, and we tumbled into the grassy spot beneath our feet. A crazy lust overcame us. By the time we were back on the path, my hair was tousled, and I am sure my face was flushed. We each had a big grin on our face. We had dared convention and had followed our passion.

"Canada is a lot bigger than Denmark," I declared gleefully. "Perhaps other such amazing places await us once we are back home again."

As the years went by, we sometimes took a long weekend for ourselves. We usually headed west while the grandparents looked after the kids. Because we were young immigrants from Europe, the Canadian splendours that surrounded continuously overwhelmed us. To this day, I vividly recall happy tumbles among Rocky Mountain meadows bright with shimmering daisies.

We bought a worn-out old army tent from a friend and ventured bravely into the wilds in Banff National Park. On our first trip out we found just the right spot. Kaj had been a Boy Scout in Denmark. He efficiently set up camp close to a rushing river, gathered dead firewood and cooked supper. We hoped wild things would come walking by and go to the river to drink. When the night got chilly, we snuggled into the warmth of our blankets and giggled.

"Was that an owl hooting? Shh... I think there is a bear prowling around our camp. I heard it and I think there are mountain lions around here, too. Maybe we should have gone to a campground instead of pitching here."

We nuzzled deeper into our little nest, feeling excited, passionate, and loved.

In the morning, a park warden, dressed in typical warden gear, called us out of our tent. We were a bit puzzled. He explained to us that camping in the open was not allowed. He recognized our newness to Canada and, smiling with understanding, suggested we camp at the Tunnel Mountain campground and enjoy our stay there.

Banff is the oldest Canadian National Park, replete with mineral hot springs. After splashing in those fantastic pools, we took the gondola up Sulphur Mountain, explored the history and elegance of the Banff Springs Hotel, and hiked to wonderful new scenic panoramas. Oh yes, these were the impressive places we had looked forward to when we immigrated.

Another cup of coffee and my mind goes back to when we were a young family.

On warm weekends, we would pack up the kids, the dog, and sandwiches and drinks for a picnic, and drive into the foothills outside of Calgary. We also wanted to go family camping in British Columbia. On our first trip there, we travelled past Banff, Lake Louise, and Golden. By the time we reached Revelstoke, I was stiff with fear that we would slip over the road edge and tumble deep into the valley below. Until 1962, the Trans-Canada Highway was only a two-lane road, bending around blind curves, up high passes and down deep mountain slopes. Little wonder I imagined my entire family disappearing among the boulders and trees at the bottom of those steep canyons.

By the time we reached Sicamous, we knew we were safe. The road straightened out. With the milder temperature, tenting seemed less daunting. For the first few years, we had that old canvas tent, quilts, and blankets. However, we soon graduated to air mattresses and sleeping bags.

Our next tent was a lovely blue contraption given to us by a friend who had travelled all over Europe, where he had collected numerous badges. His wife had sewn these bright crests onto the flaps of the tent. This collection was a great conversation starter. Our family studied their origins and talked about all the wonderful places we might visit someday, too.

These little bits of colour also grabbed the interest of our fellow campers. They often came over to our campsite with comments such as, "Did you really take the children with you to all those faraway places?" or "Was it not hard to travel with the little ones such distances and then live in a tent there?"

Others talked about their own travels.

"We went to Switzerland, too. It was in 1951, but we went by boat with our two children and rented a car once we landed in Amsterdam."

On and on they chattered about their own travel experiences, and we could barely get a word in. We had only been to a few places in Europe and not with our tent and never with our children. Before we knew it, we met whole new families. In the evenings, we gathered with them around flickering campfires. Usually somebody had a guitar, and we sang our little ones to sleep. After the children were safely in dreamland, we grownups talked and laughed long into the night until the fire reduced to a gentle glow. The next day, we sometimes exchanged names and addresses with our new friends before each of us went our own way. All that because of the badges on our tent flap.

The last sip of my coffee is getting cold, but one more memory emerges, reminding me of those happy family days.

We were in Banff, shivering in the cold as our three children tried out their Christmas presents: skis. Brand new skis, and a membership in the Polar Bear Club. After New Year's, the three children began skiing in earnest.

"But Dad, we have to be in Lake Louise for the meet by nine tomorrow morning."

"Mom, please pack our lunch now. Remember, no bananas, they get squashy.... I lost my ski pass; what am I to do?"

Rush, rush, rush. We found the ski pass. I packed three lunches and two thermoses.

"Oh, where is the third one? It is probably still in the trunk of the car from the last trip. Quick, clean it.... And throw out all the wax paper, crumbs, and wipes from the backpack.... Finish packing... And don't forget the après-ski snacks.... Stop yelling! Just get on with the program."

We warmed up the car, got the kids in the back seat, stuffed all their gear into the trunk, and left in the dark, chilly, early morning hours, headed for Lake Louise.

Another snowy day of waiting at the bottom of the hill for hours, shivering and waving as the kids came down the run again and again. Their smiles and shouts were our delight as they headed up the mountain again. By four o'clock, the competitions were finally over; everybody was happy and tired. We piled into the car. By the time we reached the highway, three young people were sound asleep in the back seat. Two hours and 190 kilometres later, we arrived at home. Dad carried the littlest one into the house. I tucked the sleepy five-year-old into bed.

"We had a lovely day today, didn't we?" I asked her.

Her answer was the full day's reward, and I shall always remember it.

"Oh yes, Mommy, someday this is going to be one of the good old days."

Finally, Kaj and I collapsed into our chairs with a nightcap, also exhausted but happy.

The sun is up now, and my cup is empty, but the memories are rushing in.

Chapter 2:

The Box

She is in the box. It is a beautiful box, intricately inlaid with various kinds of wood. The box is quite small, only a little larger than a shoe box. It stands on a table covered in red velvet. A large candlestick is on one side of the box and another on the other side. By the box stands a gilded frame with the image of an elderly lady with sparkling blue eyes and a head of dark, wavy hair.

She is in that box. The minister is speaking of her life and what a wonderful wife, mother, and grandmother she had been. I sit in the pew with my father-in-law, whom I call "Dad," and the rest of the family. I wonder why I am not crying. I only feel very sorrowful. My heart fills with memories of the day the doctor diagnosed my darling mother-in-law, whom I always called "Mom," with Alzheimer's.

Just weeks before the diagnosis, Mom had finally passed her driver's license test in my car and was so proud to be able to drive to the homes of her sons. She had been a very determined lady. She had failed the written test five times but persisted and succeeded.

Shortly after that happy day, she was unable to recognize that the car keys would also open the car doors. That was the first time we, as a family, sensed that from now on Mom would need special attention and all our patience and love. I watched her physical health declining and her mental cognition progressively diminish for eleven years. We all felt that her final passing seemed a blessing.

As I look around me, confused and even angry, I ask myself, "Why are all these people here, and why are they bringing flowers and cards and lunch to this little church? Where were they all when Mom was helpless and lonely?" My throat feels parched, and my eyes are dry. I feel as though an anvil is pressing on my chest, and I can hardly breathe. However, as I close my eyes, visions of better days appear in my mind. Slowly, I realize how much I loved this woman from the first day we met.

Early in 1960, Kaj and I wanted to get married in California because my own mother lived there. I wanted her to give us her blessing. She, though, had often made it clear to me I had been an encumberment and disappointment to her all my life. She predicted this marriage to him would lead to no good end. I also was pregnant. She told us in no uncertain terms that her approval was not forthcoming. We were not welcome.

As a result, we eloped. We found a pastor in the phone book who married us in his own home two days later. We went to see Disneyland and enjoyed ourselves like children. A few days later, my new husband and I flew from California to Copenhagen to meet his side of the family in his hometown, a small village in northern Jutland.

I was quite skeptical about our reception, since in California we had experienced such a very negative response. Since we were considered to be such a pariah by my own mother, it seemed clear to me that Kaj's family would tolerate my arrival, but not receive it well. I am not a shy person, but at that first meeting I could barely open my mouth. Terror gripped me. I was among strangers in a foreign land. How would Kaj handle this awkward situation? My new "Mom," however, opened her arms to me and introduced me with pride to her large circle of family.

I was surprised. Both his parents accepted me with warmth. We were invited to many homes to eat and eat some more. Danes are well known for their splendid smorgasbords, which I enjoyed endlessly. There was one problem, though. My pregnancy was not yet far advanced, and I suffered severely from morning sickness. As a result, many of the offered delicacies ended up in the toilet. My new Mom always understood and waited for me to get better. She then took me shopping or visiting or made me rest. Slowly, I began to believe these people really were happy to see us. They showered us with gifts when we finally left to return to Canada. At least a dozen relatives waved us off with best wishes and last-minute tokens of affection. I loved Mom from the start. Though she is gone now, I still love her. Always will I carry many cherished memories with me.

During those eleven years of watching Mom decline from a radiant woman to a sorry little heap in a wheelchair, I learned to accept that there is no return to the good old days, nor any hope for recovery, when Alzheimer's strikes. I worked with special populations in my career as a recreation therapist and always admired people's doggedness to hang on to life. With Mom, it was so very different. My emotional involvement and attachment made me resent the very tenacity which kept her alive for so long. I tried hard to make her last days bright. I visited her often with Kaj. But more than that, I watched Dad stand by her side, unflinchingly loyal, without complaint.

Now I look at Dad as he sits with the rest of the family at Mom's funeral. He looks shrunken and desolate. Sixty-seven years of togetherness make breaking their bond seem cruel. They were devoted to each other. They left their homeland and followed their two sons to Canada. I wonder, "Does he look at the box of ashes, recalling the many incidents and important moments they shared? Does he remember the days so many years ago when they left everything behind to come and watch their family grow? What did he feel when, after all these years in Calgary, he had to give up their

9

apartment? Was it difficult for him to move into care with her?" Yes, they had to move into a care home together, for he had become legally blind by then and could not look after himself without her by his side. When I think of how Dad stood by her twenty-four-seven for all those years without complaint, I feel selfish.

The church empties and people go downstairs for refreshments. I continue to sit and stare at the table, the flowers, and the candles. The wretched feeling is not leaving me, and I feel abandoned and forlorn. I want to tell Mom one last time how much I love and miss her, but Mom can no longer hear me. She is in the box.

Chapter 3:

Are Memories Real?

The summer days are getting shorter and, with them, the vividness of my cherished memories of my husband. I like to remember him as extremely handsome. In his photo album, which I made for him on his fiftieth birthday, he looks very smart. I thought he became better looking as his dark hair turned to pepper and salt. Then it turned a distinguished snow white. As the years went by, though, he lost all his hair, and now I find it difficult to imagine his earlier looks.

He was six feet tall, slim, and muscular. When we stood together, we made a fine couple. Now we both look old. Not good looking old, just old. I don't really know now what is real and what is just wishful imagination.

He was the kindest, most gentle young man I had met. He was dependable; he had a clean sense of humour; he became an involved and caring father; he was a considerate but exciting lover; he was a brilliant dancer; he was a hard worker. He was everything I ever wished for in a life partner.

Really?

Kaj had no concept of money; he procrastinated; he often drank too much; he read little and then mostly the newspapers. He did not participate in the children's school activities. He did not develop any hobbies. That was the most difficult for me. Whatever would he do with his time when we retired? I had to suggest and plan and prepare everything for us. I am curious and like to explore new places, people, and activities. He was a homebody. He did not enjoy gardening. He cooked what he remembered from his childhood, but never opened a cookbook. I, however, spoiled many a meal by happily trying new recipes. Somebody once compared us to a railroad company. Kaj was the roundhouse, always staying put and making sure that all was well. I was the train that paid little attention to the tracks. I raced into the world, trying to get to the next station in record time.

Kaj had little ambition, whereas I tried to take opportunities our adopted country offered. A comfortable home, a good education for the children, travel to explore our beautiful Rocky Mountains, sports, and theatre were qualities of life I wanted to enjoy. Kaj went along and even took part happily in events once we got him involved.

An example of how this worked. In later years, after we had moved into our Lodge, we attended their Halloween party. All residents dressed up. I dressed as a colourful gypsy, but my Honey would have none of it. "It is for children," he insisted. "I'll just watch." He did not get away with that attitude. No way. I convinced him to wear his best suit. No costume, just a suit. When we arrived at the party, I pulled my trick. "Here, Darling, just put on this black mask and pretend you are my secret lover." That was a joke he could not only understand; he played his role well when people asked him what he was representing. I instigated and insisted. He went along and enjoyed himself.

It was a challenging pairing, but it worked. Did it work as well as my memories serve me? I wish I knew. I only know that I have always loved him, and he returned my love unreservedly. We hurt each other at times. He became moody and withdrew, while I raised my voice and slammed doors. We never, though, insulted each other. The fights were fair and short. Making up was the best part of these quarrels.

Fred Rogers once said to the children in his audience, "Love isn't a state of perfect caring. It is an active noun, like struggle. To love someone is to strive to accept that person exactly the way he or she is here and now." He probably also said that we should try to bring out the best in each other. I think we did.

Chapter 4:

Early Signs

W e finally retired into our "Sweet Little Nest, out there in the West." Kaj had found the lot in Salmon Arm, British Columbia, and I had been the project manager. We designed our little two-bedroom house to our specs. We made a parking space for our small motorhome, complete with full hook-up. We built a garden from scratch and designed lovely curb appeal. All was as it should be in the ideal retirement world. We were happy for nine years. Then strange things started to happen.

Kaj slowly lost interest in financial matters. He asked me to pay for things at the store till. He handed me the utility bills that came to the house, or he'd throw them out with advertisements from the mailbox. At times, he asked me for cash because he forgot how to use the automatic teller.

My husband was never much of a gardener. Other than cutting the small lawn and picking vegetables in season, he had little knowledge of trees, hedges, or flowers. Those were my domain. But now, before he finished even his minor tasks, he would stop and wander off into the house. There I would find him aimlessly surfing through TV channels, or he would be in the garage, working on the car or motorhome.

At first, it would puzzle me as Kaj's absentmindedness increased. When he exhibited symptoms usually associated with the onset of a flu or some unexplained pain, I began seriously to be worried. He became easily tired and lost interest in daily activities. I did not like it.

"Move your bloody feet!" I yelled at him as I was vacuuming around him.

"You haven't even shaved or made your bed yet. Get ready, and we'll go for a walk as soon as I am finished cleaning up the bathroom," I nagged. My temper was being tested as I continued to see these unexplained changes in him. Kaj had always taken great pride in keeping home, garden, and vehicles in top shape. Now he often acted like a recalcitrant child, and I began to treat him as such. It was not right of me, and the joy we always had in each other was diminishing rapidly. Yet he never shouted back or regaled me. He was so neutral. I would turn my back on him, feeling guilty for picking on him.

Then I had a lightbulb moment. In her last years, his mother also had changed slowly in her behaviours and demeanours. At first, we had attributed this to advancing age, because she had been in her eighties, whereas Kaj was only in his early seventies. Perhaps he was losing more of his hearing and needed new hearing aids. We had him checked, but no; he did not need new ones. His sense of humour was also declining. No longer could we settle our differences with loving comments and silly words.

We discussed the fact that his mother had behaved in similar ways and, after many years, had succumbed to Alzheimer's. Perhaps this was inherited? Perhaps? I cannot remember how Kaj reacted to this possibility, because I was ready to panic. My brain focused on all future possibilities. Anxiety showed itself as I experienced panic attacks and severe chest pains.

We went for a special appointment with our doctor, who applied the standard test given to people suspected of having dementia. What a relief. Kaj seemed to have some problem-solving difficulties, but that did not bother us. He had severe dyslexia and had always had trouble with reading. He also wore hearing aids. I had learned how to speak to him mostly face-to-face.

Was Kaj just getting old? And what was going on with me? I slept lightly and woke to Kaj's snoring. That was new to me, and so I tossed and turned in bed until I went into the guest room to get sleep. Usually, we had prepared our meals together, but now Kaj was not interested anymore. I resented his distancing, and so I left the house more and more to busy myself in the community with volunteer work. My restlessness increased to the point that our doctor prescribed antidepressants for me, and I calmed down.

From now on, would I have to live with this man who had mental problems? Would I have to take on all the responsibilities, perhaps all the driving, and if we wanted to travel with our local RV club, would I have to drive the motorhome? There was little sense in keeping the motorhome. At that point, I was past suspicion; I feared Alzheimer's was creeping into our lives, despite the results of the dementia test. We tried to adjust to these changes.

Symptoms became more intrusive. Our conversations became serious and detailed. We talked about what to expect within the next few years, because we had already experienced the road ahead with his mother. We talked about seeing our lawyer. We should update the proper papers: Power of Attorney, Living Will, Final Testament, Appointment of Executor and Financial Advisor.

Kaj never mentioned our talks again. I tried to console myself by thinking that he simply forgot, and I began living just one day at a time.

Daily living became more and more awkward. When I asked Kaj to water the flowers, he would do so indiscriminately. When he washed dishes, he washed and dried as a little boy might. Although he had always been exceedingly clean and tidy about his person, he no longer looked after his hygiene. He vacuumed everything randomly, and when halfway done, he would go out on the deck and smoke a cigarette.

Repetitions in communications became daily annoyances for me. The time came when I had to not only take on most of the ADLs—activities of daily living—for both of us, but I now also was alone in taking on all the physical and financial tasks a household demands. Slowly, all this extra effort to be patient and understanding took its toll. I particularly feared the day would come when I could no longer cope.

Chapter 5:

Cruise with Kaj

Our doctor had assured us that Kaj was healthy and of sound mind. My suspicions of his changes in personality were unfounded. I began talking about planning a cruise to Hawaii. "Let's do this while we still have the time, money and health to make a lasting memory." Kaj thought it a good idea even though he did not expand on the why or on the how we would do this.

Everything started positively. I bought new clothes for both of us. Of course, we had to have a fancy evening outfit for cocktail hours and dances under the stars. I recalled our romantic ship journey from Europe to Canada on our honeymoon and floated on dreams of romance renewal.

I packed suntan lotion, shorts and sun hats; bought our tickets; asked the neighbours to check our mail while we were away; and off we went. We flew to Vancouver to board the *M.S. Oosterdam*. Soon I realized there were some "flies in the ointment" though. Earlier on, I'd had a vague feeling of unease as I continued to notice slight changes in Kaj's behaviour. I had reasons to suspect some danger. Why was he becoming distant? Did he think the trip was costing too much? Why did he not tell me what was wrong? I did not know what it was and wished we had not booked this luxurious cruise. Now it was too late to back out of the trip.

The first fly: Did I get Kaj and me on this ship all by myself? Kaj went along without question and easily agreed to everything I instigated. After we boarded the ship, a queasy feeling rose in my stomach. This was not seasickness. This was a feeling of foreboding.

A second fly appeared. I still was so excited about the glitter and luxury on every level of the ship. But as we explored the vessel, it became obvious how much Kaj had lost his words and sense of direction. He observed everything and everybody with silence and very few comments. He did like sailing under the Lion's Gate Bridge, though. Then he lost his way searching for our cabin.

It was impossible to discuss anything in detail. Kaj responded to questions with short words, such as good, yes, it's nice, okay, right, let's do that. He could also ask brief questions such as, "What do you want to do next? Do you want to go to Happy Hour? When do we eat?"

This lack of words and constant repetition made talking difficult, not only for me but for people around us. I tried to meet new people, but when Kaj only said hello and smiled, others smiled back and moved on. With this withdrawal of social interaction, I felt isolated and lonely. It tried my patience. Soon anger replaced impatience. My dream of a sunny cruise faded quickly.

Fly three was a big one. Kaj had lost a lot of his usual sense of adventure and humour. It was so sad for me to always be the instigator of activities or adventures. He was very observant, though, and often pointed out things others missed. One day, he pointed to flying fish in the middle of the ocean, and people flocked to see them, too.

As my birthday approached, I anticipated Kaj would plan something special for the evening. He had always been very thoughtful and liked to surprise me with flowers or a date. "Have you made a reservation in the dining room for tonight, or are you planning to eat in the Coconut Lounge?" I asked early in the morning.

"No, why do we need a reservation? I like eating at the large buffet." That hurt. He had not remembered my birthday, although I had mentioned it before we left home. But Kaj went along by putting on his blazer and looking sharp while we ate at a lovely table in a small side room. There was no romantic birthday card. There was no surprise waiting in the cabin. He didn't even apologize for forgetting my birthday. I swallowed my hurt but only cuddled up to him after he went to sleep.

The next day again, no conversation about the past, present, or future. We went ashore in Lahaina and joined others in the requisite pastime of souvenir shopping. Perhaps a new cap for Kaj to show off proudly once home? No, his old cap would do. Perhaps a little pineapple-shaped pepper and saltshaker set? No, we did not need those because we already had several others. A bright tee-shirt? No, he already had plenty. New sandals? No. My whole day was spoiled.

Kaj was disagreeable and wanted to return to the ship on the next transport. We went back. I put on my swimsuit and top, left him in the cabin, went poolside, and had a stiff drink. Let him sulk. Months later, I would feel terribly guilty that I had been so impatient. But at that time, I simply did not want to recognize that he was exhibiting early symptoms of Alzheimer's.

I felt I was losing the love of my life. This ocean voyage had spoiled many of my expectations. I was becoming a companion rather than a friend or lover. When we finally got home, we had lots of pictures, but Kaj had very few memories to go along with them.

I knew the dreaded visit to the specialist was just around the corner.

Chapter 6:

The Blue Horse

All night I kept waking up, walking the floor, and trying to harness the fearful suspicions of what lay ahead. Dawn finally arrived. After we had finished breakfast, I took another cup of coffee into the living room to settle my restlessness. Kaj asked:

"Shall I do the breakfast dishes?"

"You already did them, Honey. Thanks. Are you ready to go see the doctor this morning?"

The day to see a specialist with Kaj had finally arrived.

"Why are we going to the doctor? Are you not feeling well?"

As so often, his concern about my wellbeing rather than his own health touched me once again. The recent changes in his perceptions and strange reactions to his surroundings completely escaped him.

"I'm doing just fine, Darling, but our family doctor has recommended we see Dr. Osterman and check out what causes you to be tired so often."

Many a time I had told him small lies like that, trying to protect him from thinking of the horrible things of which I had been so very fearful myself.

The appointed time was 10:30, but we were early. Kaj settled comfortably into a chair and picked up a magazine. He seemed totally oblivious to the seriousness of the upcoming meeting. I only stared at the walls. Against one wall was an arrangement of upholstered chairs. On the opposite side hung pictures of eagles sitting on bare pine treetops at a riverside. I found myself counting how many of them were sitting on the largest tree.

My nerves were very much on edge. Beads of sweat were gathering on my forehead. I realized I was crossing my legs over and over again as I squirmed in my seat. There were several certificates hanging on a wall. One, beautifully framed, read: "Geriatric Psychiatry." Were these here to assure me I was now in very knowledgeable and experienced hands?

When Dr. Osterman walked into the room, he gave me a very positive first impression. He was wearing a brown tweed jacket, open neck dress shirt, and, of all things, blue jeans. He even had white wavy hair as becomes a professor. He asked us into his office, sat down, and made pleasant conversations about seemingly everything and nothing. He asked Kaj a few simple questions, but Kaj was slow to answer. I interrupted, "Kaj is wearing hearing aids. He sometimes forgets to adjust them. Can you help him with that, and then he might be able to answer more easily?"

The doctor complied and continued to focus on Kaj, asking him more questions. Dr. Osterman had previously given the basic written and verbal tests to Kaj to assess his mental status. When Kaj could not draw a cube or remember five words after only two minutes, I was dismayed. Forever I will remember these words, even the right order: Blue, Horse, Table, Church, Ocean. As usual, I had used mnemonics and remembered: "The little blue horse stood on the table in the church by the ocean."

The next words Dr. Osterman spoke were not really surprising, but they just about knocked the wind out of me.

"Mr. Jensen, I am sad to say this, but I have to say it. Please give up your driver's license and car keys. It is no longer safe for you to drive. There are strong indicators that you are in the early stages of Alzheimer's mental deterioration."

Kaj just looked at the doctor and, without hesitation, reached into his pocket. He never even blinked, nor did he appear to recognize the seriousness of the diagnosis. "Here are the car keys, Doctor. I don't want to cause an accident."

I reacted quite differently. I closed my eyes and covered my mouth with my hands, just to prevent myself from screaming. I knew it. I knew it. I had tried to deny it, but I knew it. When I finally stared at Dr. Osterman, I could only stutter, "Alzheimer's? Alzheimers, are you sure? That is a death sentence. Doctors diagnosed his mother when she was eighty years old, and she lasted until she was ninety-two. Kaj is only seventy-two. Our family doesn't possibly have to go through all those declining stages again, do we? How can you even say that with such ease, Doctor?"

"It's not easy at all, Mrs. Jensen. It is one of the hardest moments in my consultations when I have to tell my patients and their families how this mental deterioration causes a cruel and long journey."

I tried to digest how this progressive destruction of brain cells had already influenced Kaj's life. Dr. Osterman gave Kaj the keys back, and my doomed husband handed them to me, ready to go home. He wanted to have lunch. This thing I had feared the most was now confirmed. Disbelief and consternation. I shook with resentment. Kaj and I did not deserve this. I drove the car home in a daze. Tears blinded my eyes.

We entered the front door. All looked the same, and yet everything was different. It flashed through my head how Helen Keller, who, even though she had been both totally deaf and blind since young childhood, once said, "When you resolve to keep happy, then joy shall form an invincible fortress against difficulties."

For two years already, I had resolved to stay positive and even happy, but as we stepped inside our home, there was no resolve to keep happy. There was no joy. My invincible fortress had crumbled. That day's verdict overpowered me. While Kaj went into the kitchen looking for lunch, I got sick to my stomach, stumbled to the bathroom, and threw up bitter bile.

Chapter 7:

Sunbeams

It had been half a year since the doctor had diagnosed Kaj with Alzheimer's. Such a simple sentence. Such a huge impact on our lives. With certainty, the disorder had settled into our retirement years and changed our dreams forever.

Spring had arrived, but Kaj no longer wanted to prepare the motorhome for another season. That motorhome had been such a pleasure for us. Not only had we had a fun-filled social life and seen many beautiful sights; we also made many friends in our local RV club. Little Vanguard had been just like a hobby for him. Now he no longer wanted to bother with its maintenance. We no longer packed up and headed out.

We sold it. Our friendship circle disappeared. People did not know how to interact with a man who could not hold a conversation anymore, nor respond appropriately to questions.

Weeks passed into summer. Despite my best efforts to learn to accept Kaj's nonchalance, my exasperation reached new heights. On one occasion, when Kaj would not listen to my plan to finally see our lawyer to get our legal paperwork updated, I stormed through the house, slammed the back door behind me, jumped into the car, and drove away. There was no sense of destination. I just drove and drove. As darkness slowly approached, I turned around and headed for home.

I sat in front of our home, now our house of despair. There was no way I could go in yet. The tissue box next to me was almost empty. After a while, I turned the car keys back on and slowly drove to the nearest liquor store. A four-pack of vodka cooler in hand, I checked into a small motel along the highway, threw myself across the bed, and wept bitterly. Soon, empty cooler bottles lay scattered on the floor around the bed. The vodka did not help my state of mind at all, but it did finally put me to sleep.

By morning, I woke with a stabbing headache. Through a fog, I realized the chaos I must have created. When I sheepishly walked into the house an hour later, a frantic husband and three irate children confronted me. They had rushed from out of town to answer their father's desperate phone calls. They had been ready to call the police for help to find me. I stuttered apologies and remorse. On the inside, though, I seethed. They had answered their father's call; why did they not respond to my own anguish that way?

Instead, the family told me in no uncertain terms that the time had come for me to take on my responsibilities and stop feeling sorry for myself. There was no going back. Stop struggling; summon courage. Stop being so angry. Think of others whose lives this mental deterioration also affects. Grow up. Slowly, things sorted themselves out, but I still felt unhinged.

At last, I realized I needed help. My physician was very understanding and helpful. He started me on some antidepressant medication and suggested a mild sleeping pill to help me rest and gather my strength. It wasn't much, but I calmed down somewhat.

Then, one day as we woke, bright sunbeams crossed my pillow. I rubbed my eyes, stretched, and somehow sensed this was going to be a beautiful day.

At breakfast, the television music station was on, and ABBA was playing some of our favourite songs. The coffee was hot and reviving. Since it was a warm summer morning, I had opened the patio doors, which allowed lovely scents of lilac to waft into the house. We refilled the hummingbird feeder on the deck and leisurely continued with another cup of coffee. Before I knew it, I impulsively grabbed Kaj from his chair and laughed. "Let's dance, Honey, come on, let's dance." It was a joyous moment. Kaj and I had always loved to dance, and now we were dancing again. The kitchen floor was our dance hall. We held each other close as we slowly swayed to "I Have a Dream." He was freshly shaven and smelled wonderfully spicy. We smiled and kissed. Our kitchen was quite small. That gave him an excuse to hold me extra close, and I gladly snuggled into his neck. These few steps were so familiar and comforting. Then the music stopped. Kaj poured himself another cup of coffee and casually wandered off into the living room to watch the morning news.

I floated on a cloud of beloved memories of the many special occasions we had celebrated with friends. I thought of all the exciting dances we had attended in the Danish Canadian Club; of all the dancing we did on so many Saturday nights at home with a child standing on Daddy's shoes while sharing the rhythms. As I put the breakfast dishes into the dishwasher, recollections of the many times we had danced until dawn were beating in my heart. He still loved me, and I felt warm and cherished.

The darkness that had enveloped me for so long fled that morning. For just a little while, there was a stream of light before the dark tunnel of wretchedness surrounded me again. For those few moments on that sunlit morning, I was untroubled. I knew the tunnel was still there. I also knew with certainty there would be more sunbeams along the way, if only for a few moments.

Our legal work would also get taken care of.

Chapter 8:

It's Not Easy to Die

A person becomes a caregiver in very subtle ways. At first one thinks that their loved one is having a bad day, is perhaps not feeling well or has not slept well. Over days, weeks, and then months, things change.

I noticed these changed in my husband, Kaj, a bit earlier than many wives might notice, simply because his mother had displayed the same changes over time until she finally succumbed to Alzheimer's. Now, it had been over three years since Kaj's diagnosis, and changes in his behaviours were speeding up. We had to sell the house we had built as our "little house, way out west", and moved into a supportive living apartment in another town. Things were under control once more, or so we thought. But soon, days became more and more difficult. I became suspicious and frightened.

Outside help from a day care program on Tuesdays and Fridays for two years allowed me to go for walks or get some extra sleep. Sleep was the medicine of choice for me. Oblivion was my goal. Then one day, I received the phone call that took me down.

"Kaj is becoming too disruptive," his program leader told me. "He shouts out during programs, steals cigarettes from coat pockets that hang in the hallway, and will not sit still long enough to participate in any activities."

That news was utterly too much for me. How could professionals find him too difficult in a controlled place for a few hours twice a week, and yet expect a seventy-nine-year-old woman to look after him around the clock?

Everyone, I was certain, knew I was useless as a wife and caregiver. As his spouse, I should be able to help him and keep a check on him more so than strangers could. But I could do no more. Where was I to get the energy needed to be next to him at all times, even when I went to the bathroom?

"Why, why are you not able to just sit in your chair and watch television? Why are you forever leaving the building? Why can you not sit still wherever we are? Why do you walk away from my side the moment I am not holding your hand?" He just sat and watched my antics as though I were putting on a show.

Many times, I heard people say, "Get used to it; thousands of others are going through the same thing all the time." Get over it: what does that really mean? Young people get over their first puppy love. Others get over natural disasters, injuries, losses of kin, but can one ever get over the hurt and pain that disease, illness, and old age bring? Does one ever get used to seeing a loved one go slowly down the one-way street to death which is Altzheimer's? I was not getting over it. I felt I was the victim of misfortune. Instead of letting it go, I carried my tribulation like a hair shirt: smiling on the outside but seething on the inside.

It was on a Wednesday when too much happened, too fast, and I was more than just frightened. I had come back from meeting a friend at Starbucks, and I found Kaj gone again. He often left the apartment without notice, day or night, and frequently did not know how to get home. He would approach strangers, asking them for cigarettes and matches. When they refused him, he frequently would go to the public ashtrays and dig out cigarette butts. My heart beat faster with despair; he had probably headed for the mall. I dashed down the street, hoping he was alright. Yes, I found him on a bench outside the mall, smoking a butt.

I took him home. My heart felt the pain of utter despondency. Was I never to have a moment to myself without endangering the safety of my husband? Must I always be on alert at all times and fetch him before he managed to escape out the front door? I called my younger daughter for understanding, but she answered with, "How could you let Dad dig in public ashtrays and rummage for butts? Give him ten dollars and let him buy his smokes. It's one of his few pleasures left him."

She had no idea that Kaj would smoke anywhere, in the bathroom, on the balcony, in the garage, or in the parking lot. He knew that the Lodge where we lived forbade smoking, but his urges overcame him. I had to watch his moves constantly to avoid that wrath of the management. He also had lost all concept of money values. A dollar coin looked like a quarter to him. He sat at the dining room table, where I had set a cup of various coins to divert him from wandering and smoking, and I asked him to sort them out. He stared at them and then laid them out in lines, sorting by size, not value.

A few hours later, our son phoned and asked me to forgive his sister's outburst; she had just lost a major case in court. I had barely hung up when the phone rang again when an unknown voice simply said, "There is a respite bed to Kaj available in Summerland. Have him there this afternoon with just some personal essentials." The woman's voice was cool and neutral. How could she be like that? No tone of sympathy or understanding, just a quick voice of indisputable fact before she hung up.

I lost it—totally lost it—right there on the phone. They couldn't just demand I hand him over immediately. I had to have notice. I stormed about the room after the phone calls. Before I knew what was happening, I reached for relief from the panic that rose in me. I was not thinking; I just reached for any old bottle in the cupboard where I kept the alcohol. I downed about six ounces of apricot brandy, then half a bottle of white wine. I grabbed the vial filled with Tylenol. I was to ship out my husband without warning.

I remember yelling into the phone, "I'm done, I'm done. I just can't handle this anymore." Then I swallowed several of the pills and passed out.

I cannot remember just why my head felt like bursting. I was sobbing bitterly. My nose was running, but there was no tissue around. I was lying disheveled and confused in a room that was empty and bare except for a mattress on the floor. A bright ceiling light glared down on my swollen eyes. How long had I been there? I didn't know. Then it came to me. I was in a mystery movie, locked up like a crazy woman, lost forever from all that was dear to me. I fell back asleep from exhaustion and fear.

When I came to, I was only semi-conscious, but was aware of a blinding headache and an indescribable heartache. I lay in a hospital bed with strange noises all around me. I realized I was not dead. My immediate thought was, "I can't even die. This just proves that I am incompetent and a miserable caregiver. The future will forever be bleak and dark."

I wanted to die, but I found out it is not so easy to do. I would have to learn to continue living while my husband was on a certain death spiral from which there is no escape. Nobody could tell me how much time would pass before his body would finally succumb, as his mind was dying day by day. It was this inevitability that had overwhelmed me.

Chapter 9:

Embracing Help

M any times, I have heard people say, "Get used to it; thousands of others are going through the same thing all the time. Get over it; there is nothing you can do about it." Every time I heard that, I became quite annoyed, even angry. I thought my situation was different.

Get used to it—get over it—what does that really mean? Does one ever get used to seeing a loved one slowly go down the unpaved, potholed, one-way street to oblivion because of Alzheimer's? I know many people seem to get used to it, but I do not know how they do it—or if they are just hiding or denying the truth.

What to do? I asked myself this many times but could not find an answer. Peer pressure often says that a loyal and caring wife should visit her husband in the Care Centre where he is living, at least twice a week, perhaps even daily. One of the children says, "Mom, you should go to see him only when you feel it necessary." Another child says, "Visiting might not make a difference to Dad, but the staff might pay extra attention and care when they know Mom can show up any time unexpectantly." A close friend says, "You should go on with your life and try to find some happiness." The doctors say, "Suit yourself." So what should I do?

Now, years later, I don't much care about the opinion of others. I do not have to "get used to" my problem. I don't have to "get over" my problem. I have to figure out how "to live with" this inescapable Alzheimer's situation. I have realized that my feelings of regret, remorse, abandonment, guilt, and even shame were wearing me down. I also realized that I had been trying to please others and seek their approval. I had set myself standards for how others see me instead of examining how I see myself. I felt useless; my best was not good enough. I still felt very angry sometimes. I knew anger is useless, yet I did not know how to let it go. I was wasting a lot of energy being angry, but I felt justified to be so furious.

Then came the day I had to admit that I needed help. I was not functioning well. I decided to seek professional advice and/or medication.

On the recommendation of my doctor, I took a first step. I joined a group sponsored by the local health authority. It was a special group, only for caregivers. I went every Thursday morning to the hospital for almost two years, and slowly I changed my thinking. Here we were cohorts learning how to manage our lives when our loved ones suffered from all kinds of dementia, including Alzheimer's. In this room, we sat around long tables and shared our stories. Since the facilitator assured us that everything said in this room was strictly confidential, we freely talked about our fears, our disappointments, and our coping strategies. We drank a lot of coffee and used up a lot of tissues with our tears.

These stories were mostly about feelings. We also talked a lot about the unpredictable future. Would we be able to face loneliness, abandonment, even relief? Trying to reason things out seemed useless. Instead, we were learning how to accept things we cannot change, how to develop the courage to change the things we can change, and to find the wisdom to know the difference. We had turned to the words of the Alcoholics Anonymous (AA) and Al-Anon Family Groups principles.

Slowly, I understood I was living mostly based on my emotions—these feelings which I had always tried to hide from others and from myself. I learned to read inspirational books and enjoy the daily quotations of successful people who told of their own healing tools. Then came a turning point in my life. I found my self-worth.

I had been a bundle of painful and negative emotions, but slowly I learned I can control my thoughts, formulate my choices, take action, and then acknowledge the feelings. I recalled suddenly how my supervisor at Foothills Hospital in Calgary, where I had worked with special populations many years previously, often reminded our staff, "When assessing a patient and scheduling recreational and therapeutic programs, keep five things in mind. Apply these five A's to your programming. What is your patient's Awareness, Attitude, Ability, Accessibility, and Affordability?"

I became my own patient who wanted to change my own mental and emotional condition. I recognized a lot of my abilities and affordability, but I also recognized that my attitude still needed a lot of adjustment. As yet, I had not explored the many supports that were accessible to me. There was a lot of work to be done before I could actually learn how to "live with it."

Chapter 10:

It's Not Easy to Live

When I woke on a thin mattress on a hard floor with one stark light source shining down on me in the hospital, I realized I had failed in my attempt to die.

"I can't do this anymore! I'm done! I'm done!" I cried out as tears poured down my cheeks. As I became more conscious, I realized my personal physician was at my side. All he did was place me on suicide watch and prescribe a strong sedative that made me drowsy and listless. I wondered how he could have such a heartless approach to a desperate patient. Could he not see my despondency? A nurse gave the medicine to me, and I slept again.

Sometime later, a friendly face bent over my bed and asked if I wanted to talk about what had happened. His demeanour was so kind and reassuring, I reached out to him as though he was a lifeline. It turned out Dr. Blain was a psychiatrist and, indeed, my lifeline.

At first, in the hospital, I had no concept of time, but I vaguely remember being allowed to get out of bed and go to a small lounge where I could read old magazines or watch senseless television. There was lots of idle time in the sparsely furnished room to contemplate my future. My thoughts were not good ones. Our son came to visit from Alberta and gave me a cute teddy bear with a bright blue

39

ribbon. It was the first teddy bear I had ever received, and I was so touched, I cried. Our oldest daughter brought me chocolate and popcorn, knowing I loved those two treats. Our younger daughter phoned from Alberta, full of kind words of love.

During my hospitalization, the Health Care Region placed Kaj in respite at a care facility for three weeks while I was regaining my strength and reason. It was respite time for me, too. During those weeks, they also assigned a community nurse, Kate, to visit me in our apartment. She was a kind person. She even brought a box of tissues each time she came. She listened as I sobbed and sniffled my sorrows. She understood the paralyzing fear I had of the upcoming weeks. "What good is respite?" I asked. I felt the doctors had only revived me so I would have the strength to face Kaj's needs again.

Kate brought me a workbook called *The Changeways Clinic Core Program*, and she told me many people who studied it gained hope their life could become a lot better. When Kate came to visit, we would go over the comments I recorded in the worksheets. We talked of goal setting, stress, depression, lifestyle, thinking, social life, and how to prevent future difficulties. Between her visits, I slept for hours and hours. I walked a lot and ate little. The result was life preserving. Healing had begun.

I really do not remember details of what happened to Kaj while all this was happening with me. He had been sent home from the respite facility, and four days later, our son picked his father up and took him to Alberta for two weeks. A few weeks later, I vaguely remember staying in a motel for some time. We all hoped Kaj could cope with the help of staff at home in Athens Creek Lodge. He didn't, and I had to return to our suite. The medical system arranged another respite for four more weeks at another care home. That gave me time to find physical and emotional distance from his needs.

The Health Care Region also made appointments for me to see the kind and friendly face I remembered from the hospital. I had many sessions with Dr. Blain, psychiatrist extraordinaire as I recall him, after the hospital discharged me. In my ongoing sessions with him, I "let it all hang out" and freely cried myself dry. He listened with compassionate patience as I tried to explain my situation. He assured me I had not been suicidal, but rather, I had burnt out from the strenuous care I had provided for Kaj for so long by myself.

He explained to me that I am an intelligent and kind woman who has been through a lot. He pointed out that I had lived through a chaotic childhood and very painful teenage years. When a person has experienced such trauma, there are good reasons to react defensively and with doubt and fears, trying to always please and appease. We talked about a lot of things: endurance, hope, choices, attitudes, trust, intention, and most of all, my self-confidence.

"What can I do to change Kaj's Alzheimer's?" I asked Dr. Blain on one visit.

"Nobody, least of all loved ones, can change this horrible affliction. The lesson we all have to learn is that we, our families as well as friends and society, have to change. We all have to accept the past and strengthen ourselves for possible future stress and sorrows."

Then one day, after all his listening and my yammering, he quietly said to me, "Barbara, things will get better even more quickly if you could consider being less dramatic and more pragmatic." At home, I looked up the difference between "dramatic" and "pragmatic":

Dramatic: *theatrical, extreme, emotion, and even tragic.* Yes, I recognized that in myself.

Pragmatic: *realistic, practical, sensible, and even heartening.* Yes, that is what I wanted to be.

Dr. Blain helped me choose positive words in my thinking and talking. Things could be horrible, terrible, and even unbearable. Or things could be quite bad, disturbing, or upsetting.

The doctor recognized I had a sense of humour and encouraged me to use that to see the extremes in situations. I could survive putting Kaj into a care home. I might not survive if Kaj had to be sent to a prison camp in Cambodia. I could survive having lonely nights in our nuptial bed. I might not survive sleeping in a haystack in winter by myself.

Dr. Blain recommended I get in touch with our local caregivers support group. Now I had time to sit every Thursday in a room at the health centre across from the hospital and meet other men and women who shared their experiences and emotions with each other. Their stories of daunting challenges with loved ones who had dementia strangely attracted me. Relief set in as I realized these horrific mental disintegrations impact so many families. Their stories of despair and triumph gave me courage and resolve to learn how to live with Alzheimer's in our family. One lady had found strength from reading daily inspirational quotes. One from Lee Iacocca provided daily direction: "In times of great stress or adversity, it is always best to keep busy, to plow your anger and your energy into something positive." I learned to read inspirational books and enjoyed the daily quotations of successful people I read on a calendar a friend gave me. I went regularly for two years and learned to accept my situation in a more pragmatic way.

At the caregivers group, we learned there is a difference between shame and guilt. Mary C. Lamia, a professor at the Wright Institute in Berkley, California, wrote that shame often arouses anger. I realized my anger originated from my sense of shame, always thinking of myself, thinking I was the wrong person to be asked to carry this burden. My guilt also obsessed me. I was sure I had done something wrong. I was not patient enough. I had not tried hard enough to adjust to Kaj's idiosyncrasies.

We talked a lot about our feelings in that room. The feeling of being useless (shame) and not doing enough (guilt) for our loved ones. Wondering what will happen when these terrible diseases have had their final day. Would there be relief? Loneliness? Abandonment? Trying to reason things out seemed useless. Instead, we were learning how to accept the things we cannot change. I turned to the AA prayer: to accept, then to have courage, and finally to gain wisdom. Once I learned not to feel ashamed about my anger, I calmed down and instead concentrated on how to recover some peace and even moments of enjoyment.

Dr. Blain also reminded me to be grateful, and my faith community emphasized this. There, kind people who did not take advantage of my insecurities supported me. They pointed out that all of us feel small at times. It is when we love and do for others that we can find strength and a sense of value. We all are together in the struggles of life. Our pastor, Ken Jones, and I had several prayerful conversations. He, too, recommended I help myself. Too long had I spent thinking about and coping with my husband's illness, while neglecting to take care of my own basic needs. He encouraged me to try journaling for at least ten days and then read what I had written. "The soul needs nourishment, just like our body does; taking time for introspection can reap huge rewards," he told me. I did, and was surprised how much thankfulness for my blessings I had written down.

I began to read philosophical books, finding them to be skilled teachers. The Buddha says, "We are shaped by our thoughts; we become what we think. When the mind is pure, joy follows like a shadow that never leaves."

The Anasazi people of Arizona tell of how the Creator gave men a great gift: the gift of choice. The questions we ask have been asked by humans since they had time to think about this. Thoughtful choosing is time consuming, and it can be quite difficult. But I slowly realized I could choose "pragma" or drama. I could choose survival or defeat.

I learned the hard way to ask for and then accept help. Now I began to believe in myself and a better future: maybe I'd even enjoy family and friends again. What is most important for me is to accept that at times it is not easy to live, but none of us is ever alone. We must accept help and share our griefs.

Now I sometimes can figure out what to do. I don't always succeed, but that is all right, too. Everywhere in my hobby room, I have hung up motivating and inspiring quotes to keep me on track, such as:

"Cultivate self-compassion."

"Let go of what people think."

"Let go of the need for certainty."

"Cultivate laughter, song, and creativity."

And for me, most of all:

"Let go of anxiety as a lifestyle."

I am trying to follow excellent advice which I have taken from Brene Brown's book, *The Gifts of Imperfection*. I am slowly learning to not "get used to it" nor to "get over it." I now have tools and people that help me to "live with it," this awful Alzheimer's. All I have to do now is live one day at a time and trust myself.

I have chosen survival, and this morning, as I wrote this, I survived drinking unsweetened coffee!

Chapter 11:

Trinity - Admission

It was inevitable. Despite all efforts of keeping him at home, the day would come when I would have to prepare Kaj for admission to full-time care. There had been many challenges, but the major problem was that he was an incurable wanderer, a victim to his restless legs that took him down unrecognizable paths, both day and night. Our doctor assured me I would not have to wait much longer until there would be space for Kaj's care.

Then the phone call finally came.

"Mrs. Jensen, please have Mr. Jensen's personal effects packed, and bring him to my office before noon today." I was shocked and had a hard time to keep from crying. Trinity Care Centre had a room available for him, and I should have him ready as soon as possible. I was shaking.

Shortly after, I received another phone call from Trinity, and was told I could bring him in the following day. A short reprieve.

The next day began with my making breakfast as usual. I told Kaj, who had been in respite just three months earlier, that he would go back to Trinity again and visit with the kind nurses there. His reaction puzzled me. Calmly, he watched as I pulled shirts, pants, and other clothing out of his closet and began packing a small suitcase for him. For me, each piece of his things became a symbol of "separation forever." He, however, did not seem to connect the packing with going away. When I got him and his bag into the car, he thought he was just going for a car ride. I had not told him I was going to leave him.

The Trinity Care Centre is a facility with a great reputation. A smiling nurse took him with her to show him his new room. I had to stay with the admission clerk and sign papers which would keep him there—forever. My hand shook uncontrollably; my stomach churned. I was sure I was betraying his trust. Was I doing the right thing? Would he demand to come home with me?

Thankfully, another kind nurse saw my distress and helped me leave the building, while others occupied him in another part of the establishment. I made it home in the car, but as soon as I reached our—now my—apartment, I broke into shivering and sobbing.

I tried to console myself by recalling how lovely a place Kaj's new home actually was. He had his own bathroom with a sink and toilet; the staff would also provide him with help for weekly showers or baths. Each of the seventy residents had their own room and could walk anytime to any place their feet or wheelchairs would take them within the facility.

The front lobby had a huge television, soft leather furniture, and large windows that looked to the street. The centre room also had a wall of ceiling-to-floor windows that opened to the central garden. Here, residents could visit large shade trees, pleasant patios, and gardens anytime they wanted fresh air or to entertain visitors in the pleasant gazebo. A large activity room offered many pursuits. The director, Anna, had been there since the building had opened in 1997. It provided endless varieties of entertainment and opportunities for residents to explore their own interests. A library, craft supplies, and even computer access were available to all.

46

Most importantly for Kaj's safety, the doors to the outside were locked and opened only with codes. Should he try to leave while people were coming or going, he always wore a wristband which immediately alerted staff of his attempt, and they would stop his escape. Once I overheard, as I was leaving and he tried to follow, "Kaj, you have to stay here. Remember? We need you to help us count how many people have come in. Come, tell Lorraine how many you have already counted."

These respectful and kind redirections of the staff assured me that Kay now was part of a new family.

None of this helped my disposition that first day, though. I felt hollow and afraid of trying to cope on my own. To know that from now on I could no longer care for him, and that Trinity Care Centre would be a much better environment for him than our apartment, broke my heart. After dinner in the dining room, alone, I threw myself onto his bed, breathed in his smell, and stared up at the ceiling. He was gone. He was alive, but he was gone. Alzheimer's had taken away our intimacy, our friendship, and our dreams.

I remembered the ending of the movie *Gone With the Wind*. Alzheimer's, symbolized by Brett, told me in no uncertain terms, *"Frankly, my dear, I don't give a damn."*

To which I tried to have the courage Scarlett showed when she replied, while weeping on the stairs, *"I'll think about it tomorrow. After all, tomorrow is another day."*

Chapter 12:

Forlorn - The Day After

The clock showed 8:30 a.m. How was it possible I could sleep the whole night through and awaken undisturbed so late in the morning? Something must be wrong. I jumped out of bed, worrying that Kaj had again taken off to nowhere in his pajamas.

Immediately I began to panic as I ran out to our balcony that overlooks the nearby park. Maybe he had gone out there to sneak a forbidden cigarette. He was not there either. Then I remembered. He was gone. He was not in our home, but in his new home at Trinity Care Lodge.

I staggered to the couch and buried my face in my trembling hands. I had signed my dear husband away permanently. From now on, he was in the care of professionals who would look after him and his progressively deteriorating dementia for the rest of his life. What an incredible realization. I was now an Alzheimer's widow. Oh yes, nurses would allow me to see him after an adjustment period of at least ten days, but from then on, short visits would become the norm. No longer would I be the one to look after his comforts and routines. Other would look to his health and safety, but would they be able to give him moments of joy and delight? I doubted it. After all, fifty-five years of marriage do give you insight into each other's needs and desires.

Now I had to look reality in the face. I went into his room and looking around. His bed would be forever empty. I would have to get rid of it. I would have to spend the next few days packing and emptying his room. I took a final look and closed the door behind me. There are no words for the emptiness and hollow feelings that overwhelmed me.

My long Alzheimer's widow journey had begun. Had I known that Kaj's journey into mental oblivion would last years and years, I might have taken all those prescription pills still left over and ended my own life right then and there. Instead, I sluggishly dressed and went to the dining room. The concern others tried to show me sounded trite. What did they know, anyhow? They, too, had many losses, but they knew what came after their loss. I did not know and only feared that I was at the beginning of a very long and lonely journey. I had no appetite, so I ate sparingly and quickly excused myself.

Back in our, should I now say, my apartment, I turned on the television and, of all things, watched Dr. Phil. He always seemed to find answers to so many difficult problems. At that moment, though, I thought him to be a charlatan. Even he could not help a woman who had given up on her husband because he had a long-term affliction. I punched out the remote and blankly stared at the black screen.

We had gone through so much together, and this was to be our reward. Bitterness and self-loathing churned in my mind. A sense of having broken the promises I made the day we married left a bitter taste in my mouth. I had vowed to be at his side for better or for worse. I had easily enjoyed the better; yet, here I was, negating the worse. Entitlement fought with guilt.

This sense of prerogative and resentment suddenly reminded me of my grandmother. Her husband died when he was eighty years old. After his funeral, she told me, "I feel so angry. How could he leave me like this? I am now to alone. My own father died at fifty-three, whereas we shared fifty-three years of a wonderful marriage.

I should feel thankful for all those years. Instead, I am very angry at him for leaving me."

The universality of it all did not take away my forlornness, but at least I knew I was not alone in my sorrow. I also felt betrayed. Our three children did not call or come to see me. It was only much later I understood they stayed away on purpose, to give me time to sort things out.

Going for walks had often been a release for me as Kaj descended further into Alzheimer's. Usually, I had taken him with me with the hope he would tire enough to stay put in his recliner once we were home again; too tired to wander off once more. When my mind was befuddled and I felt weakness in all my joints, I knew going for a walk and sitting on a bench in the park next door would help me gather my strength.

This time, with the help of my trusty walker, I slowly made it past the park and around the block once more. Parents were picking up their children from the school nearby. Laughter and happy shouts filled the air. Life was going on around me, but I was not part of it. I felt exhausted. At last, I got back home, stretched out on Kaj's bed, and fell asleep. Concerned staff called me at six o'clock for dinner. I asked them to bring me a tray. The tray went back to the kitchen, hardly touched.

The television was now my new evening companion. It did all the talking, and I did all the listening. Somehow, that was not right. I turned it off, turned on some classical music, randomly picked up a book, and began to read. To this day, I have no idea what I heard or read or when I went to sleep. The one thing I remember is that I woke on my own bed the next morning, still dressed.

PART TWO:

RESILIENCE

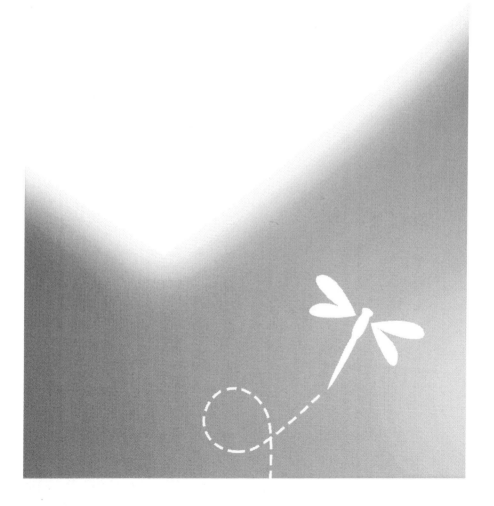

Chapter 13:

Learning to be Alone

The first days after leaving Kaj at Trinity were some of the loneliest I have ever experienced in my life. I did not open the door again to his room for at least two weeks afterwards. When I finally entered his room, I sat on his bed and looked around. I would have to remove all his clothing, get rid of the extra furniture and part with his personal belongings.

I opened the closet door. His fragrance filled my nostrils and tears filled my eyes as I laid out his remaining shirts, pants, and suits on the bed. I had forgotten to get any bags or boxes. I hurt, literally hurt. My head pulsed with stabbing pain, and my stomach churned as though I had eaten something foul. Despite the physical agony, I began to focus on the chore ahead. How to get rid of all his possessions? Would our son want things that hung on the wall? The ancient clock from his grandfather's office from Denmark? Our son did not smoke a pipe, but would he like to have his father's pipe collection? What would be of sentimental value to the girls? It all was too much to think about. I left the room, sobbing. A few days later, loaded with bags and boxes, I began to sort my husband's belongings.

In a small suitcase, I packed items for his new home first: his favourite leisure shirts and pants, underwear, socks and sandals; his shaving stuff and toothbrush. Yes, I had left him at the care home without any personal grooming items. The care staff had assured me, however, that the care home would supply those needs until I returned. His aftershave lingered in all his belongings. Never will I smell it again, anywhere, without this yearning rising in me.

For some reason, I took his best suit and hung it in my own closet. It still hangs there, and I cannot seem to part with it. When I touch it, I recall touching him. Then my mind can quickly transport me to special events when he dressed up. I recall graduation ceremonies of the children; special birthday or anniversary parties; nights when we danced away the hours at the Danish-Canadian Club. I shall leave his suit hanging in my closet for a little time longer.

I bagged the items that might interest the family and put them in the storage room. I packed up one of my quilts, some of his knickknacks, and family pictures to take to his new home. I packed the rest of his belongings with a vengeance and fury. By the time I had carried the bags to the car and disposed of them at the second-hand store, I was exhausted. All that I still needed to do was to call the Salvation Army to pick up the bed and the rest of his bedroom furniture.

Now I had an empty room. I stood there, looked around, and finally comprehended that I was really alone. My Darling would never come home again. What to do, what to do? I decided to turn the space into my studio. A place to spread out my quilting supplies and books. Now I had space for my sewing machine, and I could leave the ironing board standing. Within two days, I had transformed the room, and I felt I was gaining some control of my new life. Suddenly I also had a lot of time on my hands.

My younger daughter sent me a quilting kit, asking me to take on a challenging task. Would I cut out the fabrics and sew the individual blocks? I laid out all the materials and soon I was lost in the beauty of the colours and all the possible combinations in which I could arrange them. Then she asked me if I couldn't please join them into a quilt cover. She would have the top layered and quilted. What a clever girl. I finished the quilt for her and felt accomplished. Within a few weeks, I searched in our local fabric stores and online for more ideas. I was alive again. In the next two years, I made five quilts and found my "groove." I had become acquainted with quilting years before through a friend in Salmon Arm.

I also signed up in a local gym and exercised during the winter months. This resulted in losing a bit of weight and gaining better health. These first three years of separation were not as sad as the ones that followed. I could still take Kaj home on Sundays, and he could make phone calls to his children. He still recognized several of our residents here at Athens Creek Lodge and even stayed to listen to music programs. As months and years passed, his condition restricted our togetherness more and more. It became essential for me to focus on my own mental and emotional health. I found keeping a body healthy is much easier than maintaining a strong and positive mind. Controlling unwanted feelings of misery is much more difficult.

Chapter 14:

The Fading Christmas

Our younger daughter had the great idea of sending her father a special animal toy for that first Christmas Kaj was at Trinity Care Centre. She remembered what a caring animal lover he was. We'd had pets in the house throughout the years. Angela went on the internet and sent him an Ageless Innovation "Joy For All Companion Pets" orange tabby cat. This lifelike furry little creature has an authentic purr that sounds and feels just like real purring. It also, like an actual cat, can open and close its eyes, lift its paw, open its mouth, and move its head and body. Due to built-in sensors, this innovative lovable little cat can respond to touch such as petting and hugging. It has won the Caregiver Friendly Award for All Companion Pets and has been featured on CBS.

That Christmas, it was the largest brightly wrapped present on the table in our suite. I decorated our apartment complete with a little tree and poinsettia bouquet. I baked Kaj's favourite Danish vanilla cookies and the brown spice cookies from his mother's recipe. He had eaten his evening meal before I picked him up at his place at Trinity Centre and brought him to my apartment. I hoped he would get into the holiday spirit. Even then, though seven years ago, at a somewhat earlier stage of Alzheimer's, Kaj made no comments on how festive our apartment was. He barely looked at the presents on the table, but sat down on the dining room chair and reached for the cookies on the plate.

"Look, Kaj, look at this huge present here. The tag says it's for you." I handed him the box expectantly. He held it on his lap. "Open it, open it, it's from Angela…. You want some help?" He slowly looked at the gift package, smiled, and handed it back to me. I slowly opened it exclaiming loudly when I saw the little creature. "Oh, look, Honey, it's a furry cat. You put a battery into its soft belly and then it moves just like a real cat. What do you think?"

He took it in his hands and moved it around. This caused the toy to move as it even elicit a little mew. I should not have asked what he thought. He simply put it on the side table. "It's dead." Then he turned to a box that had a picture of licorice on it and opened that.

So much for the cat. I donated it to Trinity Lodge. For weeks afterwards I saw a tiny little old lady cuddling the little beast, cooing and singing to it. The toy had been quite expensive. I knew our daughter had the best intentions to please her father. He, however, was not responsive to specifics anymore. The lady found a joy that he could no longer have.

I took Kaj back to Trinity, then drove home alone to my own Lodge that Christmas Eve. I knew another tradition had died for us. Now I only had our three children left. There was no extended family and our three lived far away from Penticton. Had I not had the support of the Lodge staff aa well as the friendship of the residents, I think I would again have sunk into deep depression.

I put on my nightgown, grabbed an eggnog with rum, and settled in front of the TV to watch holiday movies and sitcoms. I remember being very angry. I was angry at Alzheimer's. I was angry at all the consumerism and commercialism of the season. I was angry at the songs, the smiling faces, the visions of celebrations and reunions on the screen. I was just so angry. Then I felt lonely, so lonely. I had not felt that loneliness so strongly since the day after I had admitted Kaj to the nursing home. Poets have written rhyme, famous books have been written about lost loves, but I did not know what those words meant until I experienced this hurt of the heart myself.

Somehow, as I sat there in painful misery, a feeling of hope suddenly enveloped me. I started to realize how blessed and fortunate I truly have been over the years. I have photo albums and old 8MM film reels recording many years of Christmas of joy and delight in the circle of extended family, church, and school. The surprised faces of the children when they opened their presents. The delight we all shared when they presented their holiday plays and poems under the Christmas tree. A very German tradition was that the children had to prepare a seasonal skit, poem, or song before opening their presents on Christmas Eve. While the grandparents were alive, there were ever so many generous presents and stories of the "olden days." I also recalled the Danish tradition of dancing around the Christmas tree. The looking out the window waiting for Santa to streak across the sky to visit all the children. The warmth of flannel pyjamas, cuddles and kisses. Then the hot wine mixed with cloves and honey once the children finally went to sleep. We took the best of our respective traditions and made our own new Canadian ones. We did them with enthusiasm and joy. Once the children had grown up, they braved snow and sleet to come home for Christmas; even after we retired, they came, crossing the mountains from Alberta to BC. I began to feel fortified by those memories. I would not allow one awful Christmas to remove the Spirit of love and hope from my mind or heart. There would be other Christmases to come. They might well be better, or at least not worse.

When I finally went to bed that Christmas Eve, there were no visions of sugarplums dancing in my head. No, I just had a good cry and then a bad headache from all the memories and the rum in the eggnog. I finally went to sleep, alone, without the arms of my husband around me, whispering, *"Merry Christmas, my Darling."*

Chapter 15:

Community

Just down the hall from me lived a lady, Didi, who had lost her husband three months before. I admired the way she carried herself, and I invited her to have a glass of wine before supper.

"Nobody really understands how deep the loss of a spouse reaches into our hearts." She pointed out, "One feels as though life could not possibly go on. When Walter suddenly died, I could not even cry; I was too shocked." Didi pulled out a tissue. "I carry these all the time now. There are moments when grief just hits me like a smack on the back. I find I cannot hold back the tears then."

We had another glass of wine as we commiserated. Then we went down to dinner together. Her sudden loss and my lingering separation were different, yet there were fundamental similarities. We agreed that having to become totally self-reliant was time-consuming and lonely. We had to create new ways to carry on. Didi was impressed with the way I had refurnished the second room and set it up for my quilting hobby. She invited me to her place, and when I entered, I was awed.

Didi was a knitter, crocheter, and painter. Nobody in the Lodge had commented on her talents, so it was a big surprise to see the results of her work. She had organized her shelves with baskets of brightly coloured wool and had filled stacks of containers with all kinds of tools, paints, magazines, books, and patterns.

"I have six grandchildren," she proudly pointed out. "They all love my sweaters and socks. I also knit for our church bazaar and the Women's Shelter. The painting is just for my own diversion. I am not very good at it, but I love mixing colours and even the smell of the paint."

This amazing woman was a real inspiration for me. She introduced me to her faith community.

Didi invited me to go to a Sunday service with her. What did I have to lose? Then the following week she asked me to join her in an evening group where, chapter by chapter, they had just started to share their thoughts about the book they were reading. "We've just started. Won't you join me next Thursday evening?"

I went with her and immediately felt welcome and included. I had attended many congregations during my lifetime, joined a church, left a church. This little group had established a small community of the United Church of Canada. It occupied a former furniture store. No steeple, no pews, no organ. In the foyer stood a rainbow flag and a rack of used books. It was the flag which made me feel welcome immediately, as it symbolized inclusion without prejudice. In the main room, chairs sat in a semi-circle around a small lectern backed by a large unpolished wooden cross. A piano and projector, some nice potted plants, and a large row of crystal bowls on a table completed the sanctuary. Adjoining this room were a small children's room, a kitchen, a pastor's study, and an extensive library. In the library, a dozen chairs surrounded a large table. There, people met and studied the mysteries of historic prophets, philosophers, and the Bible.

I had never been to a faith group that did not insist on a specific doctrine before. I sat down with Didi as one person lighted a small candle in the middle of the table. After a short meditation, we opened our books. I sat with amazement as various people took turns speaking about how St. Francis of Assisi's life and how his teachings affected them. They talked of the impact the book they were reading was having on them. *Eager to Love: The Alternative way of Francis of Assisi*, by Richard Rohr. He is a Franciscan priest with an unusual world view. He also has a presence on the internet, offering readings and meditations.

A young lady of about twenty with delicate features and large brown eyes began. "As I grew up, I lived in several foster homes, along with other children. I never felt I belonged. My parents are dead now and I have no siblings. One family that fed and sheltered me was very religious. The result was that we had very strict rules. Church every Sunday and many chores every day. Never did I feel valued, let alone wanted. My prayers were fervent, but God never answered. Despite these obstacles, I kept seeking God's love, but I was confused and lonely." She paused, then continued. "Since the last meeting, I read in this book that we cannot find God 'out there' until God is first found 'in here' within ourselves. Instead of asking for forgiveness or strength, I have now learned to pray, 'Who are You, O God, and who am I?'"

After she finished speaking, I sat in wonder.

An elderly man then spoke up. He looked tired in his old, worn-out suit. "I am an alcoholic. I have been dry for over ten years. I went to countless Alcoholics Anonymous meetings during that time and believed in a Higher Power. This belief carried me, but it never made me happy." He sighed heavily, then resumed his story.

"I was surviving, not living. I began to study the history of religion throughout the ages. The horrors that have been perpetuated over the centuries, in the name of prophets, appalled me. I was so disturbed to think God would permit these atrocities that I gave up on the Higher Power and began drinking again.

"I came here accidentally and have stayed. It took some courage, but I continued seeking. Slowly, I have sensed that I truly am part of it all: the neighbourhood, my country, the planet, the universe. Then I remembered that, as a child, I was told God is everywhere and always knows what I am thinking and doing. At that time, I had perceived God as an old man who looked down from heaven; loved and ruled us all. But now I understand. I have God in me, and therefore, I also have the power to rule myself. I have the Love of God in me, love for myself and for all others. I am thankful for all I have and for all the people who have helped me. I have begun to live."

As this man finished speaking, his words were sinking deep into my mind and heart. "Are these words an answer to my unhappiness?" I wondered.

Our group finished studying the book's 13 chapters over a three-month period. Before Easter, we observed Lent. I had previously thought it a foolish church calendar thing, but now discovered that a bit of self discipline goes a long way. We also had fun with pizza nights in winter. On summer Sundays, we gathered for group picnics in the park. We operated a small food bank, assisted in several community projects, and celebrated traditional holidays. Our group accepted everybody, regardless of belief, status, orientation, gender, or age. Nobody was turned out or judged. I was never asked my denomination or doctrinal beliefs; only told I was welcome.

Now I have a belief that nourishes and sustains me. While the pandemic has meant I cannot meet with this loving group, I am content to have found a community without borders, that offers unconditional love, even hope.

My friend at the Lodge, Didi, also showed me that doing for others can be rewarding, but one must also learn to live alone. After all, what are the alternatives? Becoming bitter and hard and never being happy again? I'd had enough unhappiness the last seven years. It was time to practice self-love and reach out with compassion to others. I had to learn and believe that I am never alone. All of us are in this life together.

Chapter 16:

Dreams and Nightmares

It is the nights that hold both pleasant dreams and nightmares. Since the day my husband went into care, in my sleep I still sometimes turn toward his side of the bed and wake when my hand reaches into an empty, cold space. For fifty-five years we shared our bed, lusted, created, cried and laughed together, and slept entwined in each other's arms.

Now, seven years later, I wake alone in the wide bed. Advanced Alzheimer's had robbed me of his presence. When night descends and I turn out the lights, dreams and nightmares appear. Sometimes I have splendid dreams of how it was when we celebrated our love and affection for each other.

When I open my eyes in the dark, I often wonder: should I be happy for such bright memories, or should I feel desolate, knowing I will never, ever have that contact again?

Accepting these inevitable changes is still very difficult for me. Sometimes, when I cannot sleep, I rise and get a drink of water. On moonlit nights, I put on my housecoat and slippers, go out on my deck, and wait for my love to speak to me. I take my glass of water, sit in my rocking chair, and wait. Sometimes it gets chilly, and I wrap a blanket around me as I will him to talk to me. Eventually, I hear his deep voice and I feel comforted.

Once, he reminded me of how we enjoyed raising our children. Another time, he talked about how each year we made long weekend dates in the mountains just for the two of us.

"I rented that cute little cabin in the Kootenays, again," I hear him declare. "Pack up our swimsuits and hiking boots, and hope for sunny days."

During those days, we would take in all the splendour of the Rockies. We would swim in the hot pools and hike the high trails which offered fantastic vistas around every bend. That was easy to do in the four National Parks that were our backyard to Calgary. In the evenings, when we tired of our adventures, we would retreat to our little nest, eat supper, and then go outside and wait for the moon.

The moon, whether full or wane, threw shadows and eerie shapes through the branches of the trees. The meadows sparkled with white daisies in season, and the mountain ridges glowed pink with the last sunbeams of the day. During those hours, we huddled together on a rock or log with a cool Molson beer or a hot mug of tea and savoured the mysteries of the night. At times, a deer or moose would silently step out of the shadows, look at us, and then disappear into the underbrush. It was then that we often talked about earlier years. He would chuckle as he recalled the time we spent the first camping weekend together: the wet tent, the chilly rain, the Coleman stove that ran out of fuel. Yet, we laughed as we called to mind that misadventure.

"Remember the old fur coat inside the sleeping bag that warmed us when everything else was wet and cold?" Kaj asked.

We had to giggle at that memory, and then we made passionate love. It was wonderful.

On another full moon night, a dream was so real. I will remember it for a long time. The man was tall, dark, and very handsome. His blue eyes shone like stars. He wore old-fashioned pleated trousers and a plaid shirt open at the collar. As he came near, he smelled of gasoline and automobile fumes with small undertones of Old Spice lotion. He had a small smudge of grease on his clean-shaven face.

"You want to come with me?" He invited, "Come for a ride in my yellow Lincoln hardtop convertible. We could have lunch in Banff and look at the bears at the town dump."

A strange warmth enveloped me. This attraction to him surprised me, since I had never gone out with a man who so easily assumed I would go out of town alone with him. Yet, I did get into his car. The car suddenly lifted off the ground, and we flew over the foothills into the Rocky Mountains and circled like eagles above Banff. I saw the Banff School of Fine Arts below us, then Sulphur Mountain sparkling in the sunshine. Suddenly, we landed in a meadow below Tunnel Mountain. I saw a picnic spread out on the grass. We feasted on tuna sandwiches and apples. Soon we became happily lethargic in the warm afternoon sun. As we lay back on the blanket, he looked deep into my eyes and asked, " I really want to kiss you, badly, may I?"

Before I could answer, he brushed my lips with a gentle but insistent kiss.

"Who are you to think you can kiss me?" I breathlessly replied.

Abruptly, I awoke in my bed and wondered why my blankets were kicked off and I was breathing heavily. I reached for him and then realized this stranger in my dream had been my future husband.

"Why did you leave me?" I cried. "We should have flown back home to Calgary."

Now the only thing that was real was my lying alone here in my bed with a beautiful memory. These precious dreams don't come often.

Instead, I wake in a sweat when a nightmare occurs. Strangely enough, I usually dream in colour, but when the nightmares come, I see them in black and white and sepia shades. They bring strange versions of my Darling getting confused as he wanders outside our building and gets lost in strange places. In these nightmares, I lose him in Denmark. I lose him in Portugal. I try calling to him to stay away from ledges and tall buildings to avoid falling. Then I wake. I suddenly sit up, perspiring and feeling utterly helpless. I have the feeling something is chasing me, and I cannot run away; the sensation that I keep losing things and cannot find them; the icy fear of falling into a black hole; the thought that Kaj would cry out for me and I could not hear him. All these repeat themselves and leave me sleepless for hours. During these sleepless hours, I relive the reality of the last twelve years.

The lovely dreams which I wait to emerge seldom ever do. The nightmares sometimes continue, though. I spend those nights tossing and turning in the empty bed until morning, unless there is a visible moon shining. Then I go through the routine of standing on my deck with bittersweet hope in my heart and wait for that well-known voice that tells me again that our love is forever.

Chapter 17:

The Photo Album

Over the next four years, I regularly visited my husband, Kaj, in the Assisted Living home where he lives. Usually, I would see him twice a week, and would either take him for a car ride or bring something familiar from our past. These visits were both satisfying and yet quite taxing. On the one hand, I was always so pleased to see that the staff cared well for him, and that he seemed quite relaxed. On the other hand, I was visiting a man who once had been a wonderful husband and father, but now was a tired and confused old man: a victim of Alzheimer's.

One time when I visited Kaj, I brought our old brown photo album with me. I guess because it caught me up in my own happy memories, I thought it would do the same for him. But he was living only in the present. Pictures of his childhood in Denmark did not interest him, nor did pictures of his new life in Canada. I put the album aside and continued sitting with him, waiting for him to start speaking.

Kaj smiled crookedly at me in his familiar way. I felt my heart warm as I held his hand. This hand, that had touched me in every tender and loving way for years, was now gnarled and speckled with many brown spots. They were his hands, though, and I felt connected and cherished. I began to ask some simple questions.

"When you were a little boy, your father built you a bicycle, right?"

He nodded and replied, "We got good kids. When are they coming to see me?"

I explained to him they could not come until the snow melted on the mountain highways in the spring.

"What month is this?" he asked, and when I told him it was January, he said, "They got snow tires, so they should come now."

Then I asked him whether he ever needed snow tires in Denmark.

He lost his train of thought and replied, "We got good kids. You come again on Wednesday, okay?"

I get so exasperated when that happens. I never know whether he actually understands what I am trying to say.

His primary care aide, who is a wonderful lady, passed by and he shouted at her, "Come meet my wife!" Kaj is severely deaf and mostly speaks at top volume. Of course, she had known me for nearly four years by then, but we introduced ourselves again as usual and knew he was glad we met. And then he explained to me that Cathy was going to get married and go to Ireland on her honeymoon. His perception of time was out of kilter. Cathy had married and returned from her honeymoon eight months earlier.

Once more, I tried to get a concrete answer from him. "Did you enjoy lunch today?"

However, he answered he wanted me to come on Wednesday, and so it went on for half an hour as he began "sundowning." This phenomenon is also known as "late-day confusion." It saps my patience that this condition is so progressively debilitating.

Kaj still had a sense of humour, though, which he exhibited on another visit. Usually, he sits in a very comfortable recliner in front of the television in the lobby. One day, I teased him a bit. "You are always sitting in this beautiful chair. Is it yours? Did you buy it?"

"Nope." He chuckled and grinned. "I leased it."

Another time, while I was taking him for his weekly car ride around Skaha Lake, I questioned him about his children, how many he has, what their names are, and if he is proud of them. He named all three of them and assured me, "They are good kids."

But then I asked him, "So you have three wonderful children. Do you also have three wonderful wives?"

"No." He sat up a little straighter in his seat, pointed his gnarly finger at me, and softly exclaimed, "Only you!" When he said that, I realized again that love crosses many borders.

Recently, when I came to visit, instead of walking up to Kaj, I waited for him to see me first. Sure enough, as he looked up from the television, he called me by name and had the happiest smile on his face.

"Come see my room. It is over this way." Kaj got up from his favourite chair and, taking my hand, proceeded to lead me throughout the building. He explained to me where the activity room was; where he played bingo and brain games; the cage with a budgie chirping; the large dining room; the daily menu; and the television in the lounge. By the time he had proudly given me the entire tour, he took me by the hand again and said, "Come see my room; it is over this way." We took the entire tour again, and by then he was ready to sit and watch TV. I left.

For about two years, I usually went to the local mental health centre once a week to take part in a support group for those who have a loved one who suffers from dementia and now lives in care. I learned to understand the patience required to sit with the loved one and try to communicate. My heartache and sorrows go deep into my soul. My longing for things to get better is always there, even though logically I know for certain that improvement is impossible and there is only a slow spiral toward death. In the many months and years of this process, I have found the sundowning the most onerous. To see Kaj slowly become more and more confused is hard to endure. Then I leave him with the wonderful skills of his care team, and I slip away, gratefully eased from some of the tension each visit creates.

A short way down the road is a pub. I sometimes go there after a visit and try to relax over a cool beer and fries. I attempt to focus my mind on how great it is that Kaj is so at ease in his new home. That his home is a haven for him and that he suffers no pain or stress. That for me it is easy to reach him my car in ten minutes from my own apartment. But although I have been practicing positive thinking and hope to always find something good in inevitably sad circumstances, I still find it a very difficult undertaking.

Chapter 18:

Then Came Missy

People often ask me, "How do you enjoy living in a retirement lodge? You get two good meals served every day. You have weekly housecleaning and have your sheets and towels washed for you. Supportive living accommodations must be a sweet deal."

I only say, "No."

We had known for some time that Alzheimer's would dictate how we would spend the rest of our retirement years. Shortly after his diagnosis, my husband Kaj's idiosyncrasies had become unmanageable. The time had come to sell our house and move into Athens Creek Lodge. It was not a sweet deal. It was a comfortable necessity. I feel fortunate that we could live in this beautiful place. However, we had lived here only two and a half years before I had to surrender the love of my life to a full care facility. We have now lived apart for several years, and since then I have often felt desperately alone.

Tears, depression, and a debilitating anguish sometimes have overwhelmed me. Never had we been apart during fifty-five years of marriage. The first year we were away from each other was the most painful. Sure, I now was independent and had great supportive services. But that did not alter my feelings of anger and self-pity. I had moved Kaj's recliner into his little room at Trinity Care Centre. Now I sat forsaken in my own recliner by myself forever.

I slowly adjusted to this inevitable situation. Finally, I realized I could do something about it. Gradually I took an interest in my physical health, joined a walking group, and went swimming at the public pool. I took part in the activities that are offered at my Lodge. I went to my faith community and joined a book club. Still, my heart would not heal.

Then, some time ago, an article appeared in our local newspaper that caught my eye. The story of a ten-year-old cat that the SPCA had rescued touched my heart. She had the good fortune of having received extensive care there. She was healthy and now looking for a loving permanent home.

When I went to see her, her gentleness immediately captivated me. At that moment, I realized that for me to be well and whole again, I had to have twenty-four-hour companionship. I had to be responsible for the care of another living being. I adopted her that very day. She and I have become two old ladies who love and console each other.

A new lifestyle emerged. Missie quickly established a healthy routine for me. I had to get up each morning to her gentle coaxing. Some mornings, I even woke with anticipation of what this new day would bring.

Then a spring morning came, which brought me a happiness I thought I would never feel again. I woke to the soft meowing of Missie. But instead of turning over for a last snooze, a familiar fragrance of spring tickled my nostrils. I sneezed with delight. The lilac in our old home also had this powerful scent each spring. Instead of sorrowing for the days gone by, I stretched, got up, made coffee, and fed Missie. Then I took my mug out on the deck, sat in my rocking chair and enjoyed the freshness of the scented morning.

The day was a soft blue with feathery small clouds drifting along. I had to get my sunglasses. Missie lay at my feet with half-closed eyes.

"This is the life," she seemed to purr.

I agreed. I was in no hurry. The meteorologist had predicted a warm day, and I took full advantage of the morning coolness.

An hour later, I decided to get moving. I showered, dressed, and headed out to the park for my morning walk. Laughing children were leaving the playground and heading into their classes. I felt delighted that I had the freedom to stay outside. In the park, a huge red chestnut tree was in full bloom. Birds twittered in the bushes nearby. I sat down on my walker and took in this astonishing beauty.

Suddenly, I remembered I had not eaten breakfast. My stomach turned me homeward, where I made my favourite toast with peanut butter and honey, cut up an orange, and enjoyed these out on the deck.

My senses were acute that morning. For the first time in a long time, I had seen, smelled, and heard everything around me with a clarity that amazed me. I felt wonderful. It had been a most extraordinary morning. I know my little black cat had given me the key to this newfound bliss.

On most mornings now, I first sit in my soft rocking chair out on the deck to watch the sun rise. I reminisce about the many times Kaj and I watched glowing sunrises on our travels. Then Missie leaps on my lap, and I chat about everything and nothing, past and present, while she purrs her agreement.

Soon after my refreshing morning walks, Missie meows for her daily brushing. I am pleased she enjoys all my care. My craving to be needed and wanted is well served.

On inclement weather days, I have the good excuse to watch the news on Channel 4. I do not understand most politicians, ministers, or comics. Somehow, these three careers seem to constitute the news these days. Then it feels good to have a comfortable recliner and sit with my friend on my lap as we watch even the gravest news reports. When she vibrates with her contented purrs, I imagine she is telling me not to worry about the big world, but to just enjoy our little circle of life.

Chapter 19:

Shoulder

It was spring again when I received a phone call from a very kind nurse at Trinity.

"I'm sorry to tell you, we found Kaj on the floor this morning. Apparently, he had fallen during the night behind his chair. He was bleeding from his wrist and scalp. When we tried to pick him up, he screamed out in pain. Slowly, we were able to raise him into his bed. It appeared obvious he had broken his shoulder. Then we called the ambulance."

The news shocked me. I could not quite grasp the situation. I always expected a call from the Care Centre to tell me he had died.

They told me how the ambulance had arrived within minutes and transported him to the nearby hospital. Kaj needed x-rays for a possible fracture. My heart seemed to stop for a minute.

"When can I see him? What can I do? Is he going to be alright?"

The very kind nurse assured me I could do nothing until the hospital returned Kaj to his room. I could wait for him there, but nobody knew how long it would be before he would be home again.

I was ill prepared for such a situation. It never occurred to me he could fall and break a bone. I found my shoes and purse and hurried to my parking spot. The pillar in the parkade was my nemesis. For years I had avoided it, but on that day the car left a green streak on the yellow pillar as I backed out. I shook with fear as I hurriedly drove to Kaj's home. Yes, after having lived in care for three years already, the care facility had become his home.

Hurry up and wait. As I sat waiting for two hours in his room, I looked around me. He had only a small room furnished with a hospital bed, a bedside stand, and a built-in desk under the window. The drawers in a highboy were labeled—one drawer for socks, one for underwear, one for pajamas, and one for his personal things like chewing gum, tissues, and some loose change. On top were pictures of the family, an empty vase, and a sippy cup half filled with apple juice. In a corner stood a low TV stand with casters and a shelf that held two pairs of shoes. I'd had his favourite recliner brought here from our home, but he never sat in it. The chair, instead, was a collector for extra blankets and throws. I had hung a homemade quilt on the wall over his bed, but the room still looked sparse. Old greeting cards covered the corkboard on the wall. Many of them featured pictures of dogs. People seemed to remember that Kaj had always had a favourite dog. He loved dogs. He did have his own little bathroom, but no shower. How were they going to give him his weekly shower when he had broken bones?

I cleared the blankets off the chair and waited for Kaj to be returned. When the ambulance brought him back from the hospital, the staff confirmed he had, indeed, broken his left shoulder. The nurses eased him from gurney to bed, almost unconscious but alive. I shivered when I saw his bleeding hands—his broken shoulder had been covered; I dared not touch it for fear of hurting him. Could this accident not have been avoided? But I knew it could not. One of the many reasons he had to live at Trinity was because he was an unpredictable wanderer. Night, day, it did not matter; he had to get up and walk off without knowing where he was going. Of course, he could eventually lose his balance and fall.

On this bright May morning, Kaj lay in his shadowed room, covered only with a sheet and a light blanket. It was one of those woven hospital blankets which do not warm one very much. Kaj's silver hair was rumpled; his hands were covered in blue and green bruises; his beautiful blue eyes were dim and unfocused; his skin was pale and cold to the touch. Care aides had cut a tee-shirt open and covered his chest so that he at least looked partially dressed. Staff had pulled up a railing and had stuffed pillows under his legs so he would not attempt to get up again.

What could I do for him? Offer the apple juice with a straw? Whisper loving words to him? Did he even know I was at his side? I was at a loss. What could the staff tell me other than that they had found him on the floor, bleeding and unconscious? Would he need surgery? No, the shoulder would have to heal on its own. He could wear a sling and take painkillers as he requested, that was all. His bruised hands would be alright.

From then on, he was bedridden for six weeks. At last, Kaj became more alert. He wanted only two things.

"I want ice cream, vanilla ice cream," he muttered again and again. "Will we get ice cream for dinner? I want vanilla ice cream."

He usually whispered this to me as soon as I arrived. Sometimes, I would bring him little ice cream cups and feed him. He then would become more animated and give me a weak smile. Was this his way of letting me know he still trusted me to bring good things into his life?

The other thing he wanted from me was that we establish a schedule for my visits. Obviously, Kaj now felt most comfortable with predictable routines.

"See you on Wednesday," he said each Sunday as soon as I walked into the room.

"See you on Sunday," he repeated each Wednesday as soon as he saw me.

Was this Kaj's way of letting me know he missed me? Or was it just repeated nonsense? He could not talk about any specific thing. He never, ever complained about anything, either, whereas I was ready to pick a fight. A sense of helplessness often causes anger, and I was mad—in fact, enraged and furious. Helplessly, I watched as this condition crippled his mind and wasted his body. Days on end, I sat with him, held his hand through the protective railings. I prayed endlessly that the medical profession would continue to keep him comfortable with loving care.

During those weeks and months after Kaj broke his shoulder, I lost a lot of sleep. I had not yet learned to walk into his world when I visited him, then walk back into my own where I could enjoy my quilting and my social connections. Even when I went on a trip to Hawaii with my daughter, I still carried the yearning for my life partner around with me. It took many more months before guilt left me whenever I had enjoyable experiences without him.

Chapter 20:

Ice Cream

S ummer came and went.

Kaj could finally stand up but not walk on his own anymore. Because he had become so very weak, he had to use a wheelchair. His biggest treat was to go for a car ride. This was a big job for me now. Staff policy forbade giving help beyond the entrance door. I had to drive the car as close to that door as possible and then more Kaj from his wheelchair to the front seat of the car. He is much taller and heavier than I am; therefore, that short transfer was always quite precarious. Once I got him strapped in, though, I could drive him to Okanagan Falls for his ice cream treat at Tickleberry's.

On one such day, I had become quite exasperated. Over and over, Kaj had repeated nonsensical phrases. At long last I yelled at him, "I love you more than any person on earth... so why are you driving me crazy? Can't you just quit repeating yourself all the time?"

Kaj just looked ahead, but then put his hand on my knee and very quietly said, "I love you, too."

Never will I forget that amazing moment. He might be unable to converse with me anymore, but he still could touch my heart with his love.

Time went by and our visits continued. Usually they were short— fifteen to twenty minutes. Nonetheless, by the time I drove home, I usually was exhausted.

Kaj's hearing aids had broken over time because he would not keep them in his ears. He tried to "fix" them all the time, taking batteries and filters out and losing those. Then he would go into the nursing station without permission and attempt to find new ones. People had to lean close to his left ear and shout slowly at him. This effort, together with his lack of comprehension, created a vast distance between us.

Yet, whenever I entered Trinity and saw this wrinkled old man sitting quietly, hunched over and looking at the floor or staring into space, I became heartsick again.

He had been six feet tall with wonderful sky-blue eyes and dark, wavy hair. He had enchanted my young heart. His gaze had lifted me into dreams that might actually come true, and they mostly did. For fifty-five years, he had been a husband, a lover, a friend, the father of our three children, and much more. We laughed and cried at the ups and downs that life threw at us, but we always had each other's back.

Can I really bear seeing this man shrinking into a little skeleton, with eyes now empty and a mind with little grasp on reality? Yes, I can. Do I have to learn to live gracefully with the fact that he will eventually die in his room at Trinity? Yes, I do. What other options have I? Sometimes there are still precious moments when we can smile together, hold hands, and kiss until a next time. Those exceptional flashes of awareness give me strength to carry on patiently in our strange marriage in a new and deeper way than I could ever have imagined. No matter the changes, he still is the love of my life. He looks up and still recognizes me, smiles, and waits for a kiss. A kiss that always was only ours. Or, was he maybe wanting more ice cream?

Chapter 21:

He Spoke

It is autumn again, and as I sit with my usual coffee on my balcony, wrapped in my warm housecoat and a blanket, a most unusual day from the past came to mind.

It had been a hot summer day. Temperatures had risen close to forty degrees Celsius and most people sat around air-conditioners or lolled at the lake. The unfortunate ones sweltered in the heat, listless, seeking shade wherever possible. I was lucky. I had air-conditioning at home and in my car, so I drove to Trinity to see my husband.

He sat in shorts in his wheelchair and smiled when he saw me. "I want to go outside," were his first words as I arrived. I barely had him out the door into the garden when he began to reminisce about life in Durup, his hometown village in Denmark. "We had a garden where Mother picked vegetables. Brother John watched and then he peed on the herbs; I think it was chives. I don't like chives when they're put on potatoes. I always think of John."

What amazed me was that Kaj spoke in full sentences as he recalled this childhood event. He continued, "When I had my motorbike, I went to the beer pub in the next town. Some friends were there. I drove home. It was getting dark. I heard a bump. My bike fell over and I did too. I had hit a dog. She died a few days later.

She had puppies before she died. My Dad made me pay for the dog. I did not mind. I am so sad that the puppies did not have a mother."

He paused, sitting quietly in retrospection; then carried on for over ten minutes. I held his cold hands in mine and waited. It had been so long since Kaj even spoke one complete sentence; yet here he was, telling stories of his past long ago as if he was talking to his children. The stories had content. Kaj had spoken of love, kindness, sadness, humour and actual experienced memories. I loved it. His deep voice had been silent for months and months. Now I heard it again.

He continued, "We always went to the ocean in the summer. We took our bikes. The water was salty. Mom and Dad taught us how to swim. It was hot, like today. I got sunburned." He kept on talking as we sat under the shady tree in his garden. That this hot day brought back memories of childhood summer days astonished me. Suddenly, he stopped. A glazed look came over his face as he stared at the flowers in a pot. He had gone into the mysterious world of the unknown again.

I wheeled him back into the cool building and told Andrea, one of the staff, what he had done. She said he did this quite often. He did not need an audience; rather, he would think aloud of past incidents that seemed important to him at that moment.

"Ask him some questions about his early years. As you suggested years ago, use humour to get him going," Andrea said.

I did, and it worked. "You taught your cat good manners; what did you teach her?" I asked as I smiled at him.

"I used to sit on the table by the window when Mother cooked. My cat sat with me. I whispered to her, 'Don't say hell, damn, Jesus, bastard and such. They are bad words and good people shouldn't say those words.'"

Mother heard me. She boxed my ears. She laughed. "And don't you forget it either," she said.

I thought to ask him about his later years as a teenager. There was no response. Then I asked him why he came to Canada when he was only twenty, even though he spoke no English.

"Brother John lived in Calgary. I had no money for the taxi. I worked for Modern Motors and learned to speak English. I read comic books and went to night school. I lived with John. I went to California and got married."

"Really, did you find a good wife there?" I joked. We had met in Calgary the year before going to California, and I thought he would catch the subtlety of where he had found his wife. He did not. But then he looked up at me and made actual eye contact.

"Are you my wife?" My eyes clouded over as tears gathered. Did he recognize me now?

"Well, I would like to be your wife," I grinned.

"Sure, I think you are my wife."

Kaj had spoken only in short sentences, but he still could speak. I was delighted. I was also puzzled that he never complained about anything. He had said little about people other than, "That Trump is no good. He's gotta go." Kaj had always been interested in politics, but now he only recalled that President Trump was no good. Before I left that day, he asked me to buy him some gum. I promised I would return with gum and also some licorice candy, which he always liked.

That visit took place before Covid-19 shut down all visitations. I have seen little of him in the nearly two years since then. It hurts. Kaj is non-verbal now; he does not recognize me anymore. He either lies in bed or sits in his wheelchair, staring at the floor. He still feeds himself when in the dining room but is beginning to skip meals. He has lost weight. I have lost him.

Chapter 22:

Colours

Fairy tales usually end with "and they lived happily ever after."
For children, publishers often print these stories in books with
lovely coloured pictures that illustrate the tales. Stories in real life
do not work that way. They may start with "Long, long ago…" or "I
remember…" but also include "I wish I could forget that time…."
They mostly end without the "happily ever after." Instead, they
often end in the telling of permanent grief, helpless surrender, and
even death. There are few pretty pictures.

My own tales are stories that tell how Alzheimer's has influenced
my life. They tell of pain and how I faced it. They tell of what I have
learned about picking up the broken pieces of my life and how I put
them together again.

I like to remember happy moments, and a colour or a pattern
in nature will frequently trigger them. As a quilter, I am very much
aware of colours, their shades, values, tones, intensity, and their
relationship to each other. A certain colour will remind me of the
wonderful instances Kaj and I have shared over the years. I then
can create bright and cheerful pictures that express the joyous and
touching times of happiness in our marriage.

Sixty-two years have passed since Kaj and I wed, and my colours in quilt projects and stories have changed. Now, shadows and clouds, even dark storms, cross the clear skies on the patchwork quilt of our lives together. That is perfectly acceptable.

Without shades of grey, there could be no movement in a picture. Even black sometimes is required to give punch to a creation. Only my limits of imagination restrict my crafting something out of fabric or other medium. It is so with these stories I write. It is through colour that I call up memories. I take a colour, a pattern, a texture, and all kinds of shapes that I see at a moment, and I work them into stories.

One particular memory came to me as I sat with a mug of hot coffee on my favourite chair outside on my deck on a late autumn day. I watched the last few brown leaves quiver on the bare trees in the park next door. The skeletal branches reached black tentacles into the bleak grey sky, matching my dark mood of depression. It had taken me more than an hour to get out of bed. My muscles hurt, my bones felt brittle and old. My macular degeneration blocked my central vision. My patient cat, though, had purred at my bedside and begged me to get up.

While I sipped on my coffee, I realized I must, somehow, accept the grey and black in my life as an artist would. Though my nerves quivered like those last leaves, I focused on finding a bright colour among the dark shadows of my loneliness, and I tried to recall a memory that would cheer me up.

I looked back five years when Kaj still could enjoy a car ride around Skaha Lake to get some ice cream at Tickleberry's in Okanagan Falls. He always wanted vanilla, pure white, whereas I tried out the many-coloured flavours that were offered. Then we would take our treats and park lakeside under the willow trees. By then, he could not get out of the car without help; therefore, I would open the car doors and let the breeze blow through. The wind swayed the large willow branches like huge, bright green beards on friendly giants. Then I was happy. I am glad I enjoyed those small moments. They became rarer and rarer as the months went by. Soon Kaj was in a wheelchair, and before long, our car rides ended.

The most difficult year in which to use colours to paint my memories positively was in 2020 when COVID-19 brought everything to a crashing halt. Kaj could have only me as his designated visitor. First, I had my temperature taken at his front door. Then an object that looked like a gun was pointed straight at my forehead. Finally, I had to answer a barrage of questions, disinfect my hands, and step into a small garden room. There I had to stay six feet away from him and wear a face mask.

Kaj was stone deaf and far advanced in his dementia. He did not know who I was. We could not talk to each other at all. Staff had attempted to arrange Facetime for us, but Kaj could not comprehend that technology, so he became restless and rolled his wheelchair out of the room.

The only picture I can envision of that day is of muted, soft colours one can find on a foggy, soggy seaside day as the tide recedes. Those muted pastels could match the gentle care he had received from his care home family for the last eight years. He was fading away into another world. I visited him only twice that year. Each time was very painful for me, but I knew he was content.

There are no heroes, no quests, no bright colours, no happy ending in the stories here. Instead, the ending will be when Alzheimer's has done its last deed. The only happy tales are those I choose to create in my memories. When colours fail me, I can always turn to classic black and white. There are always options as long as my eyes can see.

Chapter 23:

Blue Memories

One day, as I sat in my favourite chair on my balcony with my morning coffee, the word "blue" came to me, and I thought about all the meanings of that colour.

There are bluebells, a blue sky, a blue mist, songs about the blues, and songs about bluebirds. Perhaps blue had come into my mind as I recalled how blue the eyes of my darling husband were. Everybody had often commented on those brilliant eyes.

"I can't help that," he used to laugh. "I got those eyes from my mother, so thank her."

It's true; her eyes were an astonishing almost violet blue. Yet Kaj's eyes were a sky blue, bright and usually smiling.

As the Alzheimer's progressed, his eyes lost the sheen, the brightness, and even the intensity. I can still see his smile and his humour. He recognizes me and lights up with his crooked little grin.

Whenever we got dressed up to go out, he would wear his dark blue suit and I would proudly hold his arm. In the movie *My Fair Lady*, Eliza sang, *"I could have danced all night, I could have danced all night, and still have asked for more."* Oh, how I love that song. It encompasses not only our happy dancing, but could be a symbol of our lives together. Dancing can be so many things. Like dancing, our lives were exciting, romantic at times, and exhausting at others. But we hung in there just because we knew we were dancing to our own tune. Blue. Dancing. What is happening?

Suddenly, I think of the baby blue of the soft crib blanket of our son. Perhaps even then I could see that the blue in the blanket matched the blue of his baby eyes. Later on, in life, those eyes became the same sky blue as his father's. He, too, has that twinkle, that smile which many people have called charm.

Some more blue: blue mountain mists. We lived in Calgary, at the foot of the Rockies, and it was perfectly normal to holiday among those majestic peaks. We often went camping, and the morning mists were a soft, cool blue, fading away to display deep blue skies filled with drifting clouds at the peaks.

After we moved into our retirement home here in Penticton, we bought two blue recliners. Kaj spent many, many hours in his, watching television. He loved soccer; just watched it without knowing who was playing or where or when. I was glad that soccer could keep him in his blue chair for long periods of time. It was then I could tidy up the apartment. I could also continue with my quilting until I occasionally lost track of time. Then Kaj would interrupt me by getting up from his chair and quietly leaving the room.

The Blues. The sound of desolation and resignation. They invoked this feeling of grief, of loss, and even deception in me. How could Kaj just leave me like this? We no longer shared our thoughts, opinions, and emotions. There was no past, no future. We had no plans, no schedules, other than mealtime and bedtime. The Blues settled into my psyche. Blue had turned to grey, a dirty, smoky grey.

There is an irony here. When the doctor asked Kaj to recall five words during the decisive Alzheimer's assessment, "blue" was the first word. He did not remember it, but for years, I would recall that word under many different circumstances. Will there ever be true blue skies again?

Chapter 24:

Smiles

Long ago, I learned to put aside any expectations that Kaj might understand any conversation beyond that required to go through the activities of daily living. For years, he has been unable to remember dates, names of new people, or events. Many times, though, he recalls occasions that are now seventy-five or even eighty years old, and we have to smile at some of his stories. The staff knows them by heart, since Kaj has repeated these many times over the years he has lived at Trinity Care Centre.

He likes to recall the day his father killed his dog. Now that does not sound funny, but it was to Kaj. Not the sudden death of his beloved pet, but rather the attention it gathered. His father had the Esso dealership in their small village in Denmark. He also had his automotive shop in the backyard where little Kaj and his dog, Max, played almost daily. In those days, mechanics had a dug-out pit over which a vehicle was driven. The mechanic stepped into the pit to work on the undercarriage of the car. With typical boyish imagination, Kaj played down there in the narrow space. He tried to get Max to come down too, but the dog would not. Instead, he stood at the edge and whined. As Dad moved the car off the ramp, he did not see Max and drove right over him. The dog died immediately and consequently received a funeral. It was the days after the funeral that Kaj recalled.

The family had ceremonially buried Max in the large backyard. Then they laid out a feast for the numerous mourners, and Kaj received much sympathy. For weeks afterwards, wherever he went in the village, people invited him to have a cookie, an apple, a piece of cake, or another treat. He loves to tell how he really milked his dog's death. In these later days, the story becomes shorter and shorter, but he still tells us he got a lot of treats because his dog died.

Kaj and his brother, John, worked together for thirty years in their automotive shop in Calgary. In their childhood, they had to share a bedroom. This resulted in many shared memories, which Kaj likes to recall. Mice terrified John. One day, Kaj put a clothespin in John's shoes and laughed when John jumped up and down, screaming in fear. On the other hand, Kaj had difficulty learning to read, and John would often help him and even read bedtime stories to him. What amused them both was when Kaj would make up stories as he pretended to read. In this way, the boys giggled at the way adults carried on over trivial things. Kaj likes to tell us he was a little terror, but people loved him anyway. I believe him. He has always liked to surprise people.

During all the years Kaj worked, he always took his black lunch box. I packed lunches for over thirty years. He can still recall the day he returned from work and told me he had a present for me in his box. Expectantly, I stepped to the counter and opened it. A dead duck with shimmering feathers lay tucked in there, its head resting on its back. The family roared with glee.

I, however, jumped back in surprise and shouted, "Never will I pack your lunch again. Never!"

Kaj grabbed me around the waist, happily laughed, and exclaimed, "Of course you will. You are a great sport. I love you."

Yes, but for a while I made him empty his lunchbox before I cleaned it. Kaj tells this story again and again, with a big grin on his face. These days he tells people, "My wife hates ducks. One day I got a dead one in my lunchbox." Kaj has told this joke for years. Each year, it makes less sense than the year before.

He also tells of how he went to Copenhagen when he was a little boy and watched monkeys in the zoo there. Over the years, he frequently called his children monkeys when they acted foolishly, and he told them they might grow tails if they didn't behave. In the last few years, though, he proudly repeats to anyone who asks him, "We have good kids. We have three kids. We have good kids."

"Ice cream, I want ice cream." Always. He loves ice-cream to this day. Since the day he has been in care, I have taken him countless times to the ice-cream shop or brought him some ice cream to his home. I like it a lot, too. In years gone by, we tried to control our weight and therefore had to cut back on desserts, including this cold delight. One time we had to laugh heartily when we discovered we had been sneaking ice cream past each other for weeks. During the winter months, Calgary gets pretty cold, so we hid our treasure in the carport. Only when Kaj discovered my stash while trying to hide his own, did we decide to be honest with each other and sin together, even in little things like a Fudgesicle. To this day, I can get a smile out of him when I ask, "Where shall I hide your ice cream, Darling?"

Since the COVID-19 restrictions, I have rarely visited Kaj. I tried waving to him through the window, but he could not focus on me. When finally, a year later, family members were allowed to visit in person, we had to wear a mask at all times, stay separated six feet apart, and not touch. He and I sat across a table from each other in the beautiful private little garden room. My husband looked surprisingly healthy and very well cared for, but he did not recognize me under the mask. He did not respond appropriately to my voice. He only smiled as he reached for the candy I brought him. Then he turned his wheelchair around and left the room.

I sat for a while, holding back tears. This slow losing of him was almost unbearable. A helpless frustration rose in my chest. Would I ever be able to at least touch him, smell him, kiss him again? By now, he had been in care for eight years. How much longer was this loneliness to last? Was he as lonely as I was? I had to think positively. No, the care team was his family now. They knew how to make him comfortable and put him at ease, using a loving sense of humour.

I pulled myself together that day. Now I have learned to smile as I accept my grief. I put it into a symbolic drawer in my bedroom. Sometimes it does sneak out of the drawer at night. I let it crawl into my soul for only a few moments before returning it to its place. It must stay there as I continue to build my own independent life.

Chapter 25:

How'r You?

Every day, we meet and greet people. We make eye contact, we usually greet each other with a quick, "How'r you?" to which comes the quick reply, "Just fine, thanks, how about you?" We don't really wait for an answer, nor do we expect to get one. It is a friendly greeting in passing, that's all. Yet I find myself wishing somebody would notice I am sometimes forcing my smile.

One day I ran into a woman at our local mall whom I vaguely recognized. We almost passed each other with, "How'r you?" But then we stopped, smiling.

"Hey, Betty, how are things going? Do you time for a quick cup of coffee?" In that split second of deciding to stop, we connected and really wanted to know how each other was doing. Betty had been a neighbour of ours in Calgary, where we had spent many hours volunteering at our children's schools decades ago. I had always thought her a beautiful, vivacious woman. But now she looked entirely different. Instead of a bright smile, she just produced a small grin, making a good show of things being alright. I could tell immediately she was in dire straights.

"You look a bit piqued. I have been through some really difficult times, too. Am I right?"

Betty sighed. "Yes, my husband had a sudden stroke a few months ago and died within a week. I was left alone. I could not find a will, and with my children scattered around the world, I could not reach them."

Oh, my gosh. I had no words for her. The shock must have devastated her. My situation was so different. Whereas her husband had left her so suddenly, my husband had been confined in a facility for endless years, a victim of Alzheimer's, and I had nothing but continuing worry and grief about my Darling. Different situations, but both of us feeling so alone.

"Life is so cruel. Why?" we asked each other, and we agreed that losses of any kind are forever. All we can really do is to get through each day, one at a time.

I mentioned to her I have found people in my faith community who hold a study group on how to cope with life's many difficulties. I was so glad when she agreed to come with me to the next evening meeting. Together, we sat around a table in the study room of the community centre to study a special book, *Twelve Steps to a Compassionate Life*, by Karen Armstrong. The book has twelve chapters. We study each chapter at home for a week; then the group gathers to discuss it. When Betty and I came into the room that evening, Chapter 3 was being discussed, and the subject was perfect for both of us: "Compassion for Yourself." What a concept. We soon learned that we often are quite hard on ourselves and expect things of ourselves we would never expect of others. We treat the people we care about with patience, with love, with respect. We are forgiving and tender with them. But why do we say we're fine when we are not? Why are we so critical and impatient with ourselves?

One tall man, who was the very image of masculinity, told us about how his children died in a car accident, how his wife left him, and how he now lives in a motel after losing his job. He had been drinking too much during these dreadful months. Now he felt terribly guilty, thinking he himself caused his dilemma. He reached for the tissues on the table with trembling hands. Tears ran down his drawn cheeks as he sobbed. The entire group gathered around him, attempting to console him. We waited for his composure, then asked him, "Do you want to figure out why you are drinking?" We gave no criticism or advice; only begged him to come back to our next meeting.

When he returned the following week, he was clean shaven, a man with hope written on his face. He assured us it was our touch and total acceptance that gave him the empathy for himself which he had never even considered before. He promised he would keep coming back until we finished the book study.

During the discussion about the chapter on self-compassion, we talked about how none of us can live on just a quick "How'r You?" We agreed everybody needs to be there for one another, be alert, and notice when a person answers with the standard, "Fine, just fine."

Do we really hear it when a person answers with, "Not so good, I feel awful?" If we do hear it, do we really want to hear details? Some of us had to admit that we probably don't. Yet a kind word, a gentle smile, or a small gesture can sometimes be enough to encourage them as they keep on their journeys.

Somebody asked, "If we offered to help that person, would the help be welcome?" Maybe, maybe not. Here was irony. We need help, but we often refuse help. We help others, but many times we reject help when others offer it.

That evening, when we finished the meeting, we encouraged each other to remember we need to practice compassion for ourselves.

Betty and I met frequently after that first night at the book study until we lost touch again when she moved away to Vancouver. I never heard from her again, yet our casual greeting in the mall that day left me with the reminder to be lenient with myself.

Now, when I ask others "How'r you?", I try to pay attention and watch for the signals that might indicate "Just fine" isn't fine. I try to respond with compassion, and if I'm asked, "How'r you?" I reply honestly. And occasionally I ask myself, "How'r You?" Then I try to answer honestly with compassion to myself.

Chapter 26:

Sixty Years

For days, it had been wet and freezing: a typical February day. My mood had been terribly sad and gloomy. Instead of sitting outside in my favourite rocking chair with a hot cup of coffee and enjoying the progression of morning, I skipped that habit altogether and stayed in my bed. With the duvet wrapped around me, I felt warm and sheltered.

Finally, I got up, made my bed, and poured myself a cup of lemon ginger tea to settle my uneasy stomach. Was this depression? Seasonal affective disorder? No, just plain sorrow and pain.

Our 60th wedding anniversary was on that day. Over the years, Kaj and I had often taken a long weekend away from the family to renew our relationship. Time to talk about other things than work or family. Time to appreciate each other. Time to treat ourselves to some little luxury. Since Banff is only an hour away from Calgary, which was our home, we usually stayed in a nice hotel, luxuriated in the hot springs, and ate dinner in style. Far removed from daily obligations, these treats renewed the pleasures of our marriage. How I wished we could do this just once more.

Now I was home alone and lonely, feeling sorry for myself and neglected. I hate those feelings; therefore, I slowly began using my imagination, and hoped that my sorrow might eventually change to some kind of joy. Our caregivers' group had taught me to not only be aware of my thoughts but also that I could learn to control them.

I began, therefore, to set aside my self-pity and instead pretended that my darling husband, Kaj, was coming and taking me on a date, just as he had done so often in our early courting days.

I made a smoothie from berries, protein powder, milk, one egg and some honey, and drank that. At least that made the queasiness in my stomach go away. Then, I cleaned up my kitchen and tidied up the living room. Kaj had been a very tidy person, and I wanted to make sure he approved of my housekeeping when he came. Then I took a shower and chose one of my favourite outfits. I even picked out a beautiful set of black underwear that had been hiding in the back of the drawer. My heart began to beat with anticipation as I fixed my hair. My nails showed a few bits of chipped nail polish. No, that would not do. I quickly removed the offensive paint, sprinkled perfume on myself, and I was ready for his arrival.

Now came the hardest part. I was ready for his approval and appreciation, but of course he was not coming; he was beyond comprehension in his new home. What to do? Control my thinking and take action.

I picked myself up, got into the car, and drove to Trinity Care Centre. I saw him sitting quietly in his wheelchair. I sneaked up behind him, put my arms around him, and kissed him on his now bald head.

When he saw me, he looked up and gave me a big grin. He still recognized me. Since his hearing was just about gone, I shouted into his ear, "Where were you sixty years ago? What did you do sixty years ago?"

"I don't know," he replied.

"Where were you sixty years ago? What did you do in California sixty years ago?"

"I engaged you!" He beamed. "You smell nice."

"Thank you. Yes, you did engage me, and we got married, too, you handsome fellow. Sixty years is a long time. Do you think we should maybe get a divorce by now?"

When I said that, he snapped back his head, glared at me with a glint in his blue eyes, and loudly proclaimed, "No!"

Humour was always a special way for us to communicate and, even now, I could make him smile and laugh. That small response was a great gift from him that day. We kissed. We touched. I made love with my Darling and changed my sorrow to joy. Our sixty years of marriage had been filled with all that life has to offer. I could continue to live with all the vagaries of life and still feel I could on.

I also know the weather will turn warm, and I will again sit in my rocking chair on my balcony and drink hot coffee.

Chapter 27:

Horseback Ride

Today I woke in my nice warm bed and just lay there, remembering a vision.

I was on horseback. A very warm arm held me safely while the rhythm of the canter swayed comfortably under us. Where was I?

"You're in my arms, Darling, and we are riding over there where the sun is setting."

"Sure, and why am I on a horse with you?" My happiness puzzled me.

"We are riding through this valley because we love animals and they love us," he replied.

That made no sense at all, and yet, as I lay with eyes half closed and thinking about this vision, it came to me.

Kaj and I have ridden through life together in a lovely rhythm, facing all things together in the hills and valleys of our lives. The sunset was a prediction of things to come. Things that put an end to the first fifty years of our marriage.

.   We had finished building our dream home in Salmon Arm, complete with a basement suite for a future caregiver. We had anticipated that my walking days were numbered. The doctors had told us that in less than five years I would probably be in a wheelchair because of my weak back. We were prepared.

It certainly turned out differently. I'm still walking, but my Darling is now in a wheelchair.

Alzheimer's slowly and unobtrusively crept into our lives. At first, we could not take slight changes seriously.

Kaj struggled with finding the right words.

"Where is… that thing? I want to check the mail," he'd say.

"Do you mean the mailbox keys? Here they are," I'd reply.

"Do you want more cream or sugar in your coffee?" I'd ask.

Strangely, he'd reply, "What's his name wanted to borrow the hedge clippers."

A few months later, he began to forget things. He'd leave the house without his wallet. Let the water overflow in the kitchen sink. Come back with an empty basket after going out to pick green beans for supper.

I began having the same feeling I remember when I was ready to deliver the children. There was that urge to clean, to tidy up, to sort things out. To rearrange everything in the nursery. I had that strange feeling, and only in retrospect did I realize my psyche was preparing for a major change.

It was so with Kaj. Later on, my doctor explained I had been in denial.

Chapter 28:

Doom Scrolling

ome time ago I learned a new saying, "doom scrolling." It hit a sensitive nerve with me. I have watched a lot of television over the last few years and have become curious on the one hand and upset on the other. I was surprised when I heard that experts have studied the effects of watching bad news for hours on end each day. The repeated fascination with seeing all the challenges of the Covid-19 pandemic, the climate changes, and political shenanigans around the world can cause us to feel helpless and defenseless.

Just what I needed in my life; more bad news. As I continued learning to live my new life as an Alzheimer's wife, I had added stress by taking in the troubles of the world as well. I needed to limit my circle of influence. One day, I sat down and took some notes. How was I actually spending my time each day? How did I feel when a day was done? I surprised myself. Since then, I have made some conscious changes which have helped me feel better and stronger.

One thing I have done is to talk things over with my cat. Missie is a beautiful cat, black all over but dressed in white cheeks, gown, and paws. She looks and listens. She meows and purrs at my voice, yet she never talks back, corrects my opinions, or laughs at some of the silly things that enter my head. My morning coffee time is now spent listening to soft, mellow music while we chat. I get a lot off my chest.

I complain sometimes: "It's too hot to go outside.... The smoke from the forest tickles my throat and gives me a runny nose.... I haven't heard from the kids in more than a week. Am I the one who has to make the call all the time?... Do we always have to get canned fruit at our meals when we have orchards right outside our front doors, with branches bending to the ground loaded with peaches, apricots, pears and apples?"

Missie just looks at me with slitted eyes. I know she will never tell anyone what has been on my mind. She is my conscience. "Be thankful your home was not burned out during the wildfires.... Be glad you have not lost loved ones to Covid.... Yes, thousands of people have been displaced as weather catastrophes obliterate their entire communities, but you can be grateful our town is still safe," she gently reminds me.

Then she purrs, and adds, "It's time to quit worrying. Shrink your circle of influence. Try a little gratitude. Contribute your energies to creativity and helping others. This you must do. You know it is the only route to find peace of mind. You can do this. You can smile, give a comforting word, even joke a little to reduce tensions. Yes, you have finished making large quilts. Those are days gone by, but you can still make small quilted items for donations to your good causes. You are not young anymore. Settle back. Recall your happy memories." Missie is forever calm. Her tranquillity flows over me, and I feel soothed.

Another thing I have done is to return to the practice of mindfulness. Without taking time to watch and listen to the good things around me in my daily life, I know I would fall back into the clinical depression I fear so much. I give myself permission to reach out to others for support when I doom scroll.

My husband has now been in the nursing home for eight years. All the visits, all the outings have become impossible since Covid-19 isolated us all. I am glad he is so far advanced in his condition that he has no concept of time, events, or special occasions. I, on the other hand, can experience all that is going on around me, and if I choose, I can feel more like a lonely widow than ever before. I can feel disappointed that my eyesight is being hampered by macular degeneration. I can choose to watch more television than in the past because it is easier than reading a book. I can choose to be guilty of doom scrolling.

Or, I can choose to stop making these choices. And I have. Since I realized how negative my thinking has been, I have been making different, more positive choices.

Now, I schedule my TV hours and have become selective in my television viewing. Half an hour of morning news and weather. Dr. Phil in the afternoon. Yes, I still watch his program. It fascinates me how people willingly go public with their tragic family issues. I like Judge Judy. She is practical, has a great sense of humour, and can judge readily who is the villain and who is the victim. In the evenings, I enjoy the privately owned channels. Not only am I saved from interruptive and useless commercials, I also learn a lot from their educational programs. I never knew, for example, that all insects combined weigh more than all humans on earth. I have learned we know more about the moon and Mars than we know about the depths of our oceans. I have found out that most empires throughout the ages lasted no more than an average of three hundred years. I set my PVR for recording good movies. I love watching old TV comedies.

Another thing I have done, instead of doom scrolling, is to limit searching for information on my iPad. There is so much conflicting information and misinformation out there that I am more confused after the searches than I was before. Heck, why do I have to know what causes loss of eyesight? My optometrist has sent me to an experienced, well-trained eye surgeon who has personally examined my eyes. Why did I think I would find better information on the internet? Besides, what does it matter what the causes are; the fact is, I am slowly losing my eyesight. So, I have quit searching for solutions.

I do, however, search travel sites. Now that I do not have the energy to travel extensively anymore I sometimes dream of places I still would like to visit. I am fully vaccinated, but with the pandemic rules and restrictions constantly changing, which countries might allow me to visit next year, anyway? And I would need a travel companion. I cannot afford to pay for two tickets anywhere outside of my province. Nevertheless, I continue searching travel sites and dream on.

The seasons are changing again. Soon leaves will turn brilliant colours before drifting to the ground. Life will continue to offer its ups and downs. I will once more turn mindfully to the beauty of nature for strength and solace. That is definitely something doom scrolling cannot offer me.

Chapter 29:

Acceptance

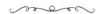

It was a crisp morning. I had to wear my cuddly housecoat to keep off the chill, as I sat with my coffee in my favourite rocking chair on my balcony to greet the day. The heat of summer had left. Fall, my favourite season, had arrived. Even as leaves fluttered to the ground, small buds were already waiting in their place for spring. As I had done so many times, I looked back over the years and recalled special days and events.

My coffee was hot. I could see the steam rise from the cup. Suddenly, uninvited tears ran down my face. I did not know the cause, but I was feeling sad; not angry or dejected, only incredibly sad—a deep feeling of painful sorrow. Just then, Missie showed up, jumped onto the coffee table next to me and nudged my hand. How did she know I was weeping? That cat often is my private little psychologist. I began to talk to her. It used to be that I chuckled at old women who talk to their cats, but now I understand it well. Where else could one unload their thoughts without fear of rejection or ridicule?

I began by telling her not to worry about my tears. It had struck me that the world was so full of contradictions. I had travelled to many places and had lived on two continents. I had seen the most awesome beauty and majesty of mountains, rivers, and seas. I had cried while hearing heavenly musical productions and had laughed outrageously at magicians and comedians. Though my early childhood had been chaotic and often cruel, I also met people during my teen years who were exceedingly kind and understanding. I had been a war child in Germany. I saw things a child should never see. My mother had somehow been emotionally destroyed by her own war experiences and, therefore, she was unable to give the loving care one usually expects from a mother. Once I came to Canada as a single young woman, my life became rich and fulfilled in adult years of marriage, motherhood, and careers. Those were decades of many challenges but also joys.

"Oh Missie, I took so much for granted. I forgot to be thankful for all the good happenings in my life. I thought the halcyon days would never end but, when Alzheimer's struck my Kaj, the world did end for me. Or so I thought.... Oh, my little pet," I whispered into her attentive ears, "Why was I not strong enough to help Kaj when he began to be difficult? Why did I become so resentful when his condition worsened, irreversibly leading toward death? Why was I so self-absorbed as not to realize that many others were going through the same thing? Most of all, how come for many years I was jealous of those who appeared to live quite a happy life while their loved one was in a care centre?"

"Oh, so now you are feeling sorry for yourself? Is that useless guilt nudging your conscience again?" Missie looked at me, purred, and then purred further: "Will you give yourself a break. You reached out for help from professionals and friends. You persisted and continued to follow all the great suggestions you have gathered from books and YouTube inspirational programs. I've watched how you progressed in developing empathy and compassion, not only for others but for yourself. I saw you when you took me for walks in the park. You were happy during those outings. I saw you newly energized when you returned from the trips you took with your children. I watched you when you were creative for hours in your quilting and painting. Most of all, I observed you when you were sleeping. No longer do you toss with nightmares. You have created a new life for yourself. You have always continued with devoted visits to Kaj and have faced all the COVID-19 restrictions."

Missie stopped purring for a moment and looked up at me thoughtfully. Then she snuggled deeper into my lap and started up once again. "So, we must continue to be strong and face any troubles which we will surely encounter. We will do so together. Remember how you told me once, 'We are never alone; even the stars are always with us.'"

I stroked Missie under her chin and scratched her behind her ears. She was a smart little cat. I blew my nose, took the empty cup back into the kitchen, washed my face, dressed, and took my trusted walker into the warming autumn morning.

Bibliography

Alzheimer Society of Canada, 5 Oct. 2021, https://alzheimer.ca/en.

Armstrong, Karen. *Twelve Steps to a Compassionate Life*. Vintage Canada, 2011.

Brown, C. Brené. *The Gifts of Imperfection: Let Go of Who You Think You're Supposed to Be and Embrace Who You Are*. Hazelden Publishing, 2010.

Chopra, Deepak. *Seven Spiritual Laws of Success*. Amber-Allen, 2007.

Dass, Ram, et al. *Still Here Embracing Aging, Changing, and Dying*. Riverhead Books, 2001.

Drew, Lorna Ellen, and Leo C. Ferrari. *Different Minds: Living with Alzheimer Disease*. Goose Lane Editions, 2005.

Mitchell, Stephen. *The Gospel According to Jesus: A New Translation and Guide to His Essential Teachings for Believers and Unbelievers*. Harper Perennial, 1997.

Newmark, Amy, and Angela Timashenka Geiger. *Chicken Soup for the Soul: Living with Alzheimer's & Other Dementias: 101 Stories of Caregiving, Coping, and Compassion.* Chicken Soup for the Soul Publishing, LLC, 2014.

Paterson, Randy J., et al. *The Changeways Clinic Core Program: Practical Strategies for Personal Change: An Introduction to the Core Program.* Changeways Clinic, 2008.

Rohr, Richard. *Eager to Love the Alternative Way of Francis of Assisi.* Franciscan Media, 2020.

Wagamese, Richard. *Embers: One Ojibway's Meditations.* Douglas & McIntyre, 2016.

About the Author

Barbara Jensen was born in 1936 in Berlin, Germany. When she was twelve years old, she immigrated to the United States with her mother. She returned to Germany after high school graduation and received her Interpreter/Translator diploma in German/English there. She came to Canada when she was twenty-one, as a secretary. Barbara met and married her husband, Kaj, in Calgary, Alberta. After raising their family for twenty-five years, Barbara received the Recreation Therapist diploma at Mount Royal College in Calgary. She worked with special populations both in Alberta and British Columbia until her retirement in 1990.

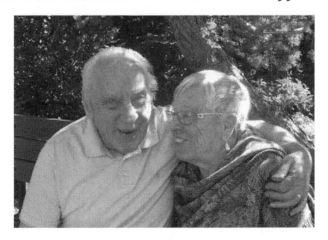

When her husband was diagnosed with Alzheimer's in 2009, she became his full-time caregiver. Barbara's memoir, *Alzheimer's Wife: A Caregiver's Journey of Endurance and Resilience*, traces the extreme frustrations and despair leading up to his admission to care in 2014; then Barbara goes on to share the many efforts and supports she sought that led her on a new journey of discovery and hope.

Gratitude

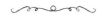

Without the encouragement of Julie Ferguson, author and photographer, I would never have even thought of writing this book. She facilitated a writers' feedback group three years ago, and all the experienced participants accepted me as an emerging writer with promise. Norma J Hill has since been my coach and editor with unfailing skill and patience. My three children, Pamela, Angela, and Ken, encouraged me to develop weekly writing habits, while my faith group and community counselling groups helped me recover after a failed suicide attempt. I also thank all the other caregivers who together shared the painful memories of loneliness and despair which many of us felt while our loved one descended into the spiral of Alzheimer's. I am indebted to those who have continued to encourage me to share my journey with other caregivers with the hope they will no longer feel alone and forgotten.

Manufactured by Amazon.ca
Bolton, ON

28306893R00079